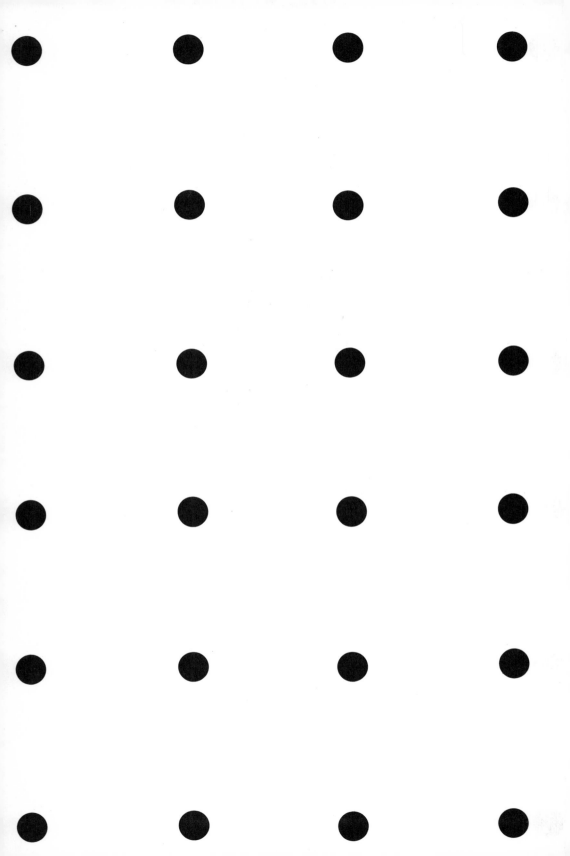

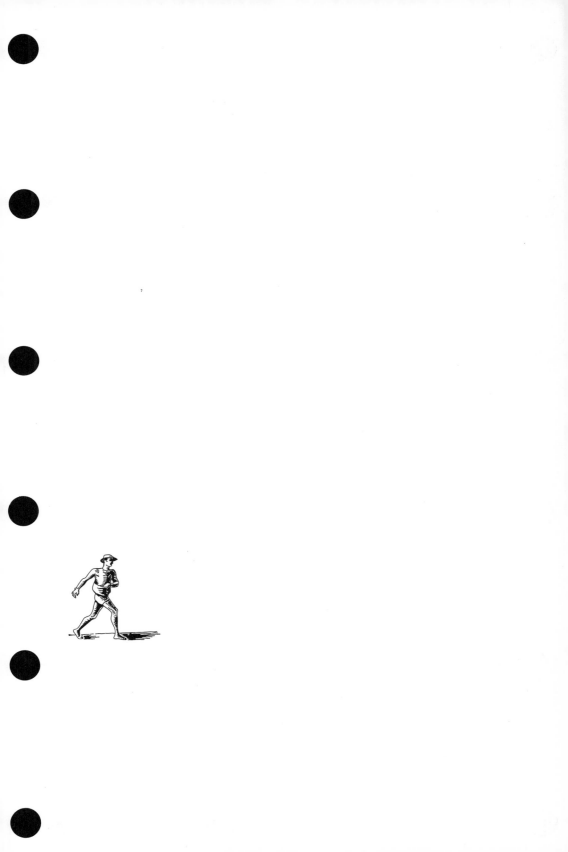

# SUCCES

•

*Effective dressing on the job,*
*at home,*
*in your community,*
*EVERYWHERE*

GLAMOUR'S®
GLAMOUR'S
GLAMOUR'S
GLAMOUR'S
GLAMOUR'S
GLAMOUR'S
GLAMOUR'S

BOOK

GLAMOUR'S
GLAMOUR'S
GLAMOUR'S
GLAMOUR'S
GLAMOUR'S
GLAMOUR'S
GLAMOUR'S
GLAMOUR'S
GLAMOUR'S
GLAMOUR'S
GLAMOUR'S
GLAMOUR'S
GLAMOUR'S

*by Barbara Coffey*
*and the Editors of Glamour*

*Simon and Schuster • New York*

Published by Simon and Schuster
A Division of Gulf & Western Corporation
Simon & Schuster Building
Rockefeller Center
1230 Avenue of the Americas
New York, New York 10020

Book design by Miki Denhof
Drawings by Durell Godfrey
Manufactured in the United States of America
1 2 3 4 5 6 7 8 9 10


Library of Congress Cataloging in Publication Data

Coffey, Barbara.
    Glamour's success book : effective dressing on the job, at home, in your
community, everywhere.

    Includes index.
    1. Clothing and dress.  I.  Glamour.  II.  Title.
TT507.C64            646'.34            79-16243
ISBN 0-671-24682-8


Photos by Rico Puhlmann, John Stember and Joshua Greene

# Dedication

This book is dedicated to women everywhere. As women, we are experiencing profound changes in our lives and in our relationship with the rest of the world. It is our hope that this book will help make the new goals now within our reach more accessible so that we can go on to yet undreamed of goals.

*The Editors*

9

# Contents

# THE BASICS

## 1
ccept your body, then
ess it effectively

## 2
How to build a good
basic wardrobe

## 3
Color: How you can
make its psychological
implications work for you

# THE POLISH

## 4
hat to wear when

## 5
How to be a good
shopper

## 6
How to organize your
closet and your clothes
thinking

## 7
he polish on your look

## 8
How to solve your
problem fashion and
beauty situations

## 9
Conclusion: Putting it
all together

# Introduction

# What would you like to be doing five or ten years from now?

Even though you may not be able to articulate precisely what it is, you probably have a pretty good idea of the direction in which you'd like to go, either professionally or personally. Whether achieving your goals takes a certain kind of education, personality, or preference for one kind of life-style over another, beginning to look as though you've *already* achieved those goals, or at least as though you're someone who *will* achieve them, can greatly increase your chances of truly succeeding several years from now. "Looking the part" is most important, especially in the early stages of reaching toward a goal.

Look at it this way. You want to sell your skills at a job and/or project a certain image in your community. Like any other product, you are judged by your packaging. Package yourself one way and you appeal to one group of buyers, package yourself another way and you appeal to an entirely different group. What's important is that you are aware of your personal packaging and the response it's getting you. One young woman's experience in this area makes the idea clear. This particular woman commutes into a large city from the suburb where she lives. She was bored with her appearance and decided it was time for some sort of change. Since frizzy curly hair was a look that was gaining popularity at the time, she decided to have a curly permanent. (Previously, she had a relatively conservative image.) The first day she had her new hairdo, she was astonished at what happened as she walked through the large metropolitan train station in the city where she worked. The conservative banker types who usually gave her an occasional admiring glance didn't give her a second look, but the more arty types were now showing approval. "I never realized how much your looks determined who paid attention to you," she said. Perhaps even more interesting was the change in the way she felt about herself. "It made me feel more available," she laughed, and I haven't felt that way in a long time; I have two small children! It also makes me want to try certain clothes that I wouldn't have thought about before." The way you put yourself together has a profound effect on how others—and you—feel about you.

We are not suggesting that there is any right or wrong way to put yourself together, only effective and ineffective ways, depending on what you want to achieve. One of the things many women are now trying to achieve is more on-the-job status.

How you look is very important. No matter how talented and able you are, dressing inappropriately and creating the wrong image will make it more difficult for you to get ahead. Conversely, dressing appropriately and conveying a certain image can be of invaluable help. This book will give you guidance for on-the-job dressing, but it doesn't stop here. All women's goals are not job-oriented. Many women don't work outside their homes, yet they have a strong desire to create an image that flows with their life goals. The working woman also has a life outside her job and she is concerned with how she looks and the impression she creates here, too.

T his book will help you make sense of all the dressing and image demands made on women today, whether you work or not, whether you live in a small, conservative town or a large, aggressive city. It will help you look your best under any circumstances, whether you are tall, short, fat or thin, or just plain average.

If you look at what's involved in successful dressing as just one more problem in a long string contemporary women must face today, it's understandable. But don't forget that the more responsibility *anyone* has—male or female—the more opportunities and options open up and the more problems there are to solve. The very fact that you now have to think carefully about *all* the images you can project is a positive thing. It wasn't too long ago that a woman had precious few images to address herself to. That's what started the whole liberation idea, and it's what makes the need for a book like this such a hopeful sign.

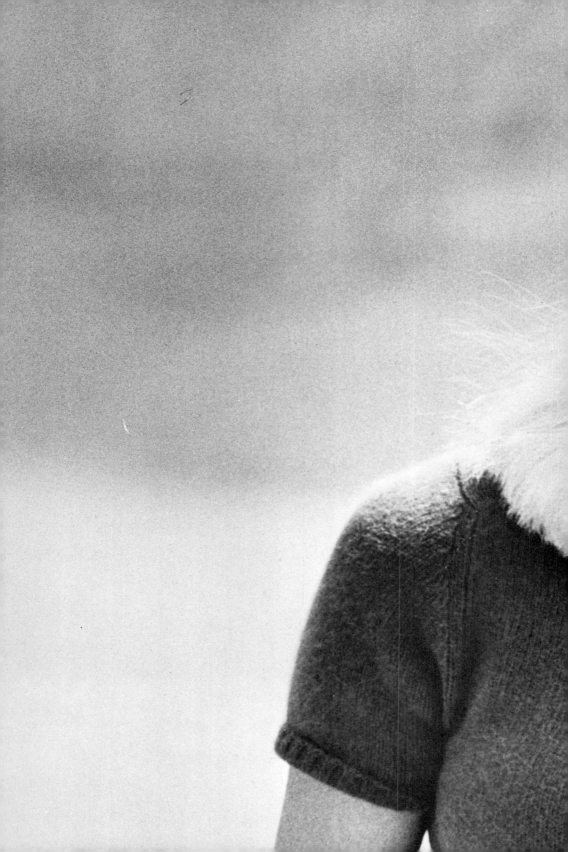

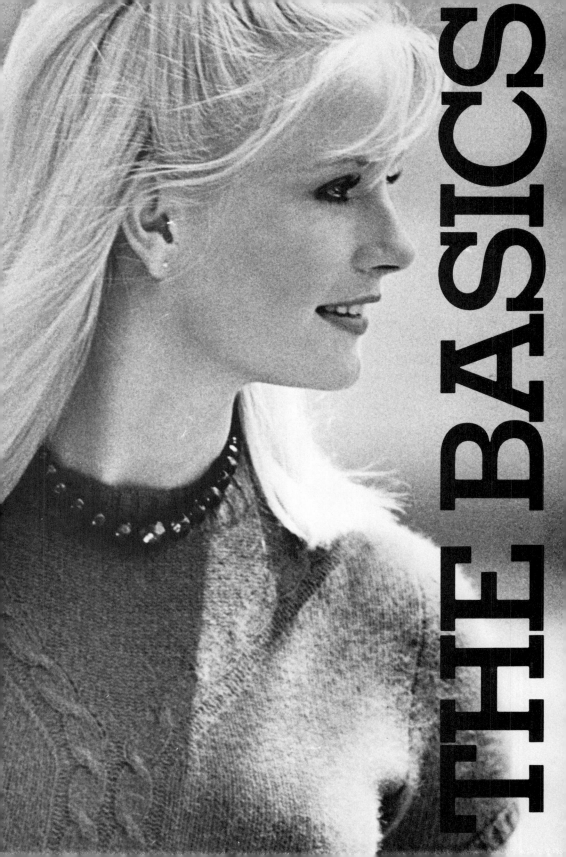

THE BASICS

# 1
# Accept your body, then dress it effectively

You have the same potential for dressing your body as effectively as the next woman. The only real trick to doing it is to know your body *objectively*. Then and only then, can you learn what looks best on you.

Although diet and exercise can reshape you to some extent, you will be short, tall, average, or whatever *all* your life. Even though you may control your weight well, its pattern of distribution will continue—if you tend to put on weight through the hips or stomach, that tendency won't change. If your shoulders are broad or narrow, if your arms are long or short, none of this will change. Now is not a minute too soon to learn what works best for whatever it is that makes you YOU. In this chapter you will find suggestions for making the most of some common body facts.

## HOW TO PUT YOURSELF TOGETHER IF YOU'RE <u>SHORT</u>

If you are one of the millions of women who are short, you know what a problem it can be to find clothes. Some things you want don't fit, some that fit don't suit you. "The choice is often between buying something that needs miles of alteration or something that fits but looks like a 'little girl going to a tea party,' " as one short woman expressed the problem. She says, "At thirty, I still felt I looked sixteen most of the time until I learned how to shop."

You will be more likely to find your fit if you learn what size range works best for you: junior, misses, or the combination size. (See pages 37 and 38 for more about this.) You should also note any stores in your area that have departments that cater to short women or carry lines of clothing made especially for them. This can save you hours of shopping time. Here are some other tips.

### A SHORT SHOPPER'S CHECKLIST

■ Shop at the beginning of the season. There's more chance of your size being in stock.
■ Check out name designers' clothes; they often come in smaller sizes such as 2 or 4.
■ Shop teen departments for good classics, such as tailored shirts and pants.
■ Try the boys' department for jeans and shirts.
■ Try French and Italian clothes; they often have a close-to-the-body cut that is good for short, small women.
■ Find a manufacturer or two whose clothes fit you and make it a point to look for this label first when you shop.

After you've narrowed down the departments and the stores that stock the best clothes for your short figure, you can help yourself even more if you look for certain things in articles you're actually considering. Here are some tips:
■ Look for clothes with simple, clean lines—they're easiest to alter and the simplicity of cut looks well on a short woman.
■ Your best coat bet is a plain reefer coat or a trench.
■ A single-breasted blazer is the best jacket shape. Check the back of the blazer carefully in a mirror to see that it doesn't look too loose or too long-waisted. These problems often become more obvious from a rear view.

■ Make sure clothes fit properly through the shoulders and neck, because of the difficulty of alteration.

■ A general guideline for hem length is just below the knee. Check your mirror and let your eye be the final judge.

■ Stay away from bulky or "big" styles: they will overwhelm you.

■ Pick small prints; big ones will dwarf you.

■ Accumulate separates rather than dresses. It will be easier to get a good fit, since dresses can pose problems at the waist.

■ When you want a dress, consider a wrap style. It does not have a definite waistline and creates no problems. A shirtwaist dress, provided you get a good fit, is also a good style.

■ Fussy details such as ruffling, scalloping, and shirring will accent your petiteness.

## Picking Accessories

Accessories are extremely important. The wrong ones can throw your look from right to "cute" or the other way round. You have to be careful of accessory size. Be suspicious of anything that on a small woman could look cute or fussy. Little plastic pins in the shape of animals or vegetables will make you look childish, not trendy. Be suspicious, too, of oversized accessories such as a large seashell pendant or a big, clunky bangle bracelet. Here are some overall guidelines to follow:

■ The best shoe heel height for everyday is a medium one.

■ Experiment with a higher heel for evening; it can give your clothes more flexibility.

■ Avoid the flattest and highest heels. Both will look wrong on you.

■ For a more elongated line, keep shoes and stockings in the same color tone as your skirt.

24

■ Try boots when you want a long, lean line.
■ Stay away from heavy or oversized jewelry. It will weigh you down.
■ When in doubt, choose the simplest, classic piece.

## The Overall Picture

Being short doesn't have to make you feel like a bonsai plant in a forest of tall pines. You can command authority, have grace and elegance. Part of the trick, of course, is believing in yourself and not letting your height make you feel uncomfortable. Here are some final tips that will help you know you're doing all the things that will make you look best.
■ Aim for a long line. Do it by keeping separates in the same color family. Keep shoes, stockings, and boots in the same color family as your skirt.
■ Don't wear strongly contrasting colors, top and bottom. A white shirt and dark skirt or pants will cut your body and emphasize your shortness.
■ Don't wear wide or conspicuous belts or choose any style of clothes with conspicuous detailing at the waist.

## HOW TO PUT YOURSELF TOGETHER IF YOU'RE TALL

If you sprouted before your classmates and learned to slouch in your seat, if you spent the first day of every school year checking the new males for tall ones, you're typical of the average tall woman who's self-conscious about her height. Whether you're aware of it or not, many women envy you. Tall women can wear clothes so beautifully; their elongated bodies help make the most of the line and cut of most styles. "I never thought of my height as a beauty asset," says one woman, "until I went shopping with a friend whom I considered average height. She picked her way through the racks of clothes exclaiming that she couldn't wear the clothes she liked best because she wasn't tall enough!'' Another tall woman says, "I knew I had something going for me when a high school friend and I wrote away to one of those modeling schools and my friend was told she shouldn't pursue a modeling career because she wasn't tall enough! From then on, I started to stand up straight and be proud of my 5' 10".

The big fashion problem for tall women is finding clothes that are long enough. One immediate solution is to take special note of shops and departments catering to you. More and more of these are appearing, many more than those catering to the short woman. If you live in an area where shopping is particularly limited, check mail-order sources. There are several good ones that sell clothes especially for tall women and for those with long, slender feet. The mail-order sections of good magazines usually feature these sources from time to time. In addition to these suggestions, here is a checklist of ideas that will help your shopping.

### A TALL SHOPPER'S CHECKLIST

■ Get acquainted with men's departments. They usually carry the look you like in pants and tailored shirts that will be cut long enough for your body.

■ Know your waist and inseam measurements and you'll be able to zero in on the right fit quickly. (The inseam measurement is the length of the inside leg seam from crotch to pantleg hem.)

■ Look for women's designer labels. These clothes are usually cut larger and have more generous hems and seams.

■ Look for dresses with no waist seam to avoid a short-waisted fit.

■ Consider wrap-style dresses. They are good choices for you.

■ Head for the tunic sweaters in the sweater department. They have the length you need.

■ Try to find turn-back cuffs on sleeves to give you an extra bit of length.

The style of any dress or put-together separates you buy should be carefully considered. No fussy, little-girl looks for you, they'll just make you look silly. You have the stature to carry off elegant, important clothes, so why not take advantage of it? You can pick things with soft lines to make you look feminine, but there's a difference between looking feminine and looking cute. It's a difference that matters to tall women. Here are some style tips.

■ Avoid fussy touches such as tiny prints, ruffles, and scallops.

■ When you buy a coat, look for a reefer, wrap, or chesterfield style.

■ Approach two-piece looks with caution. They may "split" too much and leave your midriff bare, especially when you reach up or bend over.

■ Don't be afraid to break your color scheme at the waist. A light blouse and dark skirt can keep you from looking too string-beany. A wide belt can have the same effect.

■ If you like the look of shoes, boots, or stockings in a contrasting color, wear them. You can carry off the look.

## Accessories for Tall Women

Remember to keep your accessories in proportion to your size. A small chain or pin can look "ditsy" on a tall woman. Watch out for handbag mistakes. They can be bad ones. If you've ever seen a tall woman carrying a handbag that looked as if it belonged to a child, you know what we mean. Make sure the size of any accessory you add is in keeping with the rest of your clothes and with your size in general.

## The Overall Picture

The one cardinal rule is: Don't try to hide your height. That's impossible. Instead "wear" it with pride. Don't feel you have to dress down to anyone, especially men. If the occasion demands dressy clothes, including high-heeled shoes, don't be afraid to wear them. Think of Ann and Dustin Hoffman. Even in flat shoes, she towers above him and neither seems to mind.

## HOW TO PUT YOURSELF TOGETHER IF YOU'RE OVERWEIGHT

The fact that you're carrying more pounds than you'd like doesn't mean you can't look great. One of the first things you need to do is clear your head of tired clichés that say you can't wear high-fashion clothes. Proof that manufacturers respond to women's clothing needs is indicated by the fact that there are now several lines of clothing on the market made especially for overweight women, and these clothes incorporate the same fresh styles you see in "regular" clothes.

Develop a positive attitude about your looks based on the fact that you look well because you have taken the time to learn to dress your kind of body effectively. "I used to look like a frump," says one woman. "I hated the fact that I was fat so I just didn't do anything with my looks. Consequently, I made myself look even worse. I've learned that even if I don't always discipline my eating habits, I can still look attractive and looking this way communicates self respect."

If you, like this woman, learn to put yourself together well, you'll have more confidence. Here are some tips:

SHOPPER'S CHECKLIST FOR
A HEAVY WOMAN

■ Look for good fashion. You can wear it—pick anything from a straight-leg jean to a soft romantic look.
■ Don't believe you can't wear prints or bright colors. Line and fit are more important than color.
■ Never, never buy anything that doesn't fit you, especially something that's too tight.
■ Try the misses sizes—even sizes such as 12 or 14. They're more likely to fit you than are junior sizes, 7, 9, or 11.

As you've probably gathered, ease of fit is key for you. A garment that fits well will always look better—and appear to be of higher quality—than one that doesn't. You should aim for an easy fit, one that's not loose and not tight. Finding it may mean refusing to buy some things because one size is too small and the next size is too big. If this is your problem, move on to another style no matter how much you liked the one that doesn't quite fit. Here are some guidelines:

## Good Shapes

■ Straight-leg pants (no pleats or gathers)
■ A-line skirts or dresses
■ Long-line tunics
■ Smock tops
■ Reefer or chesterfield coats
■ Wrap dresses
■ Bias rather than gathered skirts or dresses

## Good Tricks

■ Try a long scarf at your neck. It creates a long lean look.

29

■ Keep skirts, tops, stockings, and shoes in the same color family. They will elongate and slim you visually.
■ Wear a bright, flattering color. It's just as becoming to you as it is to a thinner woman.
■ Don't forget makeup and hair. Soft pretty makeup and a flattering hairstyle will attract attention to your face and away from your body.

## Picking Accessories

The old adage "less is more" applies here. Too many overweight women pile on accessories in the hope of drawing attention away from their bulk. It doesn't work, and in fact, has quite the opposite effect. Too many accessories make you look cluttered and chunkier than you really are. Think out your accessories carefully and make each piece you add serve a purpose. For example, if you decide on a long scarf, use it to lengthen your line and slim you down. Let the scarf be your most important accent. You might use a couple of strands of long beads to achieve the same effect. Remember that the gleam of gold or silver at your neck or on an arm can add a look of elegance, as long as you don't overdo it.

One common accessory mistake is picking the largest size bracelet, pin, earring, and so on to compensate for your bulk. True, you don't want to wear a tiny piece of jewelry, but you don't want the biggest, either. Pick average-sized accessories, they'll work best for you. A medium-sized handbag, a simple cuff bracelet, a pair of pretty bangles, these are all good choices.

## The Overall Picture

The one thing you should guard against is a dowdy appearance. Matronly styles and clothes that hang on you rather than fitting properly are the two main causes. If you pick the same, fresh, contemporary styles everyone else is wearing and have a positive attitude about your looks, you'll automatically appear much more attractive.

## HOW TO PUT YOURSELF TOGETHER IF YOU'RE THIN

The thin woman is the forgotten person in fashion. Most women are so busy trying to become thinner than they are that they forget there is such a thing as being too thin and that thousands of women feel self-conscious about too little weight. One such woman says, "When I was a teen-ager, I used to stuff myself with milk shakes and french fries, but I didn't gain much. I felt so sexless next to all my voluptuous classmates. I even shied away from swimming and learning to play tennis because the clothes these sports required made me so unhappy with my body."

If you're like most thin women, you probably find you look well in covered-up or layered clothing, but in more revealing things, especially summer or evening clothes, you have problems. A protruding collar bone, a thin wrist, or thin legs are most commonly complained-of. The key to finding a flattering look is to find clothes with some kind of softness to compensate for the angularity of your body. Gathers, pleats, tucks, think of all these details as your friends. But don't overindulge. Don't combine a pleated skirt *and* a pleated top—pick one or the other. Don't pick the fullest skirt, either. Too many gathers or tucks will make you look like a broomstick inside your clothes.

Be very careful about fit. You don't want clothes to be tight—that will emphasize thinness—but don't wear them so loosely they hang on you. Aim for a good fit that *skims* the body, one that definitely says there *is* a body underneath.

31

THIN SHOPPER'S CHECKLIST

■ Shop in junior departments (unless you're very long-waisted). The sizes here will fit better.

■ Try the boys' and young girls' departments for classics such as tailored pants and shirts.

■ Look for front detailing such as gathers, yokes, pleats, or ruffles.

■ Look for styles with a flounced hem, especially for evening. It's very flattering to thin legs.

■ Think of cap sleeves as a good solution for bare arms. They offer just a bit of cover over the shoulder.

■ Pick pant styles with pleats or gathers in front.

■ Avoid clingy fabrics.

■ Avoid anything with straight or angular lines or vertical stripes.

■ Consider a belted wrap coat or a cape.

## Picking Accessories

Accessories can work soft little miracles for you. They can help conceal a bony chest or wrist. For example, a low neckline that exposes your collarbone can be softened by a necklace that nestles in the hollow of your throat. A pretty cuff bracelet can hide the protruding bone in your wrist. A scarf tied softly at your neck is another good camouflage.

You need to pay particular attention to the leg area. Avoid very dark stockings; they make thin legs look thinner. Flesh-toned stockings are best for you. Remember that boots are a marvelous way to conceal thin legs and they are a great cold-weather fashion. For dressy clothes, pick a shoe with some delicacy such as a strappy sandal or a pump with a low-cut throat. Don't pick the highest heel, it isn't flattering to you. A medium heel works best. When you shop for very casual shoes, don't buy heavy-soled, heavy-heeled clunkers. They look ridiculous on thin legs. A low wedge heel or a medium, shaped heel are good here.

## The Overall Picture

Don't dwell on your thinness. Most of your friends probably envy you. Instead, put your energies into finding flattering clothes, and don't forget the softening effects of a good hairstyle, preferably one that curls softly around your face. Makeup in peach or pink tones has a softening effect while bright reds and deep wines have a harsh effect for you. One last thought: many thin women have small bosoms and this can cause a fit problem in heavier clothes such as blazers and tweedy tops and dresses. You might find it helpful to wear a very lightly padded bra under this kind of clothing.

# HOW TO PUT YOURSELF TOGETHER IF YOU HAVE A <u>FULL BOSOM</u>

In order to find your best look, you must first start with the right bra. No matter how well-chosen your clothes may be, if they're worn over a bad bra, you won't look your best. Probably nothing has changed so definitively in the past few years as have bras. New fabrics that are both light *and* supportive are the main reason. This means you'll be able to find a good bra without much trouble if you keep these things in mind:

FULL-BOSOM SHOPPER'S CHECKLIST
FOR A BRA

■ Buy in a shop that has a good fitter. Her help can be invaluable.
■ Look for reinforced bra cups; either an underneath band or wire will give the support you need.

33

■ Make sure your bra has cups that cover the bosom without binding, especially at the sides.

■ Make sure the bra band rests on your body with no wrinkling or binding.

■ Check shoulder straps; they should be substantial and not cut into your shoulder.

■ Before you make your final decision, slip a top or dress on to see what kind of line the bra gives clothes you wear.

The style of your clothes can do a lot to minimize the size of your bosom. This doesn't mean you have to spend your time in loose, dowdy clothes in dark colors. It does mean, however, that you need to be a bit choosy. Here are tips.

## FULL-BOSOM SHOPPER'S CHECKLIST FOR CLOTHES

■ Shop for clothes in misses sizes such as 8, 10, 12. This range will fit you better than junior sizes.

■ Designer clothes often have a more generous cut and could be worth the money to you.

■ Head for clothes with ungimmicky shapes that have some softness in front.

■ Pick the single-breasted coat or jacket.

■ Avoid clingy, attention-drawing knits, full peasant looks, and details such as ruffles or yokes that add too much front bulk.

■ Remember solid colors, small prints, and thin vertical stripes de-emphasize a full bosom.

■ Splashy patterns and horizontal stripes broaden.

## Picking Accessories

Remember to keep scarves and necklaces on the small side. Anything too big or flashy will only draw attention to your bosom. Try on pendant necklaces before you buy one. If the pendant hangs into your bosom, you're in trouble.

## HOW TO PUT YOURSELF TOGETHER IF YOU HAVE AN AVERAGE FIGURE

You're the lucky woman with no special problems. Good taste and clothes appropriate for the particular situation are your guidelines. You'll want to go from here to the next chapter where you'll find tips for building a good basic wardrobe.

## HOW TO PICK THE RIGHT SWIMSUIT FOR YOUR FIGURE

If you had to single out the most traumatic piece of clothing for the majority of women, it would have to be a bathing suit. Some women are so uptight about wearing one that they never appear on the beach. One woman expressed her feelings this way, "I go on a diet the month before I know I have to shop for a suit, then I stand as far away from the mirror as I can get when I try one on." You don't have to put yourself through such a trauma. Any figure can look presentable in a bathing suit if you pick the style with care. Locate your main figure problem in the group below and follow the advice given for it.

### If You Have a Big Bosom

Your first priority is good support and reasonable coverage. Suits with built-in bras can be one solution. A band under the bosom offers good support and is available in bikinis or maillot styles. Whatever the style, the fabric should be substantial enough to give you some support in

35

itself. Avoid thin, "spaghetti" straps, they don't provide enough support for your kind of figure. Be sure you check the fit from a side view. Flesh overflowing from cups can be a problem here.

## If You Have a Small Bosom

You should look for some kind of softness across the bosom, for example, gathers just below the bra cups or pleats. A suit with a design on top is also good; maybe a print or some sort of geometric design. Don't succumb to overly constructed suits with stiff inner bra cups. They will only succeed in emphasizing your problem because they look so stiff and unnatural. They also tend to make the suit stand away from your body through the bosom. There are a few suits on the market with light padding, very much like the fiber-fill used in some bras. These are flattering and present no problems.

## If You Have a Hippy Figure

A suit with a high-cut "French leg" is very flattering for you. If you don't know what this is, think of the outfits nightclub cigarette girls used to wear in old movies or the leg on a Playboy Bunny's costume. This leg cut gives a very long, flattering line that does wonders for almost any leg. Suits with adjustable hip ties which make the leg of the suit briefer are also good for you. Stay away from any suit that is binding and tight through the leg and avoid big, bulky looking boxer shorts. No matter what the style, deep colors are likely to be more flattering than pale ones.

## If You Have a Thick Waist

Look for a long, sleek line. A one-piece suit with longitudinal stripes or a longitudinal pattern would be suitable. A maillot with seaming down the sides of the front is also a good elongating choice. Two-piece suits that break at the natural waist are *not* for you. They emphasize a thick waist. A bikini is an option, but pick one that hits well below the waist. Deep colors are more slimming choices than light or bright ones.

## If You Are Overweight All Over

A one-piece suit is your best bet. Don't try to hide your weight, it's not possible; instead, "wear it well," as the saying goes. This means having enough confidence in your suit choice to forget about it after you've bought it. Check out your suit from all views to be certain that it fits well and creates no bulges you didn't have before you put it on. Believe it or not, a modified bikini is also a good choice. One that isn't too bare through the bosom and that hits you slightly below the waistline would be good. Stick to deep colors and small prints or patterns.

## If You're Short or Have Short Legs

Your best choice is a high-cut leg (more detailed description of this under hippy figure) in a one-piece or two-piece suit. A suit with a vertical pattern or stripe is another plus.

## HOW TO FIND YOUR BEST FIT*

Now that you know what sort of styles and colors will work best for your kind of body, give some thought to what size will work best. You have a choice of straight sizes, 6, 8, 10, etc., junior sizes, 3, 5, 7, etc., or what's referred to as a double-ticket size, 5/6, 7/8, 9/10, etc. If you could simply try on a few, find the one that works best, and then declare you are a size 8, 9, or 9/10, all

* From "How to Find Your Fit" by Lila Nadell, *Glamour,* September 1976.

would be well. Unfortunately, sizing is not uniform. One firm's size 10 is not the same as another's. In fact, fashion manufacturers agree that determining the measurements for their sizes is their biggest problem and often the key to their success.

A manufacturer starts the sizing process with proportions such as those in the Department of Commerce publication, "Body Measurements for Sizing of Women's Patterns and Apparel," based on a large cross section of women. These figures were last issued in 1970 and styles in ideal body shape change as much as styles in clothes. Bosoms are more—or less—emphasized. Curving derrieres are alternately desired or despised. An hourglass waist is in or out, as are shoulder pads and broad-shouldered looks.

Faced with all this, most designers rely on the dimensions of a dummy—a canvas-covered, cotton-padded papier-mâché form—whose measurements lie somewhere between the actual body and the garment to be worn over it. Although these dummies are exactingly constructed, it's possible that two manufacturers using the same form will end up with two differently sized garments. Such disparity occurs in the making of the garment. Some designers want their clothes skintight while others allow for ease over the figure.

Each designer takes the basic dummy measurements for a particular size range and varies them according to the kind of body the designer wants to appeal to. The suspicion that higher priced clothing manufacturers jiggle the size numbers is based on the fact that a designer of a better line will take a size 12 dummy and call it an 8 to flatter the customer into thinking she's a smaller size. Better clothes are not only bigger, they're also geared to a taller, 5'7" woman, ignoring the fact that 70 percent of the female population is between 5'4" and 5'5".

Finding your best fit is really a matter of trying on the same kind of garments, such as a blazer and pants, from several different manufacturers in different departments without worring about the number on the ticket. A sixteen-year-old we know thought she was a misfit as long as she shopped in the junior area. One day she happened to try on something in a young misses department and was overjoyed to find out she could be fit perfectly. On the other hand, a large thirty-three-year-old, unhappy with the "mature" styles she found in the misses department, was delighted when she discovered the on-target looks in double-ticketed styles. These double-ticketed sizes represent proportions that fall between junior sizes (which are generally shorter waisted and narrower) and misses sizes (which are longer waisted and wider). It was created by manufacturers to sell in either a junior or a misses department and may be found in both places—which doesn't make your shopping any easier.

You can narrow down your size possibilities by determining whether junior or misses sizes generally fit better, and whether you prefer the styles you're most likely to find in each of these ranges. Junior styles are usually younger looking than misses. Finally, you can note which clothing manufacturers make clothes that fit you well. When you shop, check out the styles from these manufacturers first, since they are likely to continue using the same measurements in their sizing until there is a major shift in fashion.

As you can see, finding your perfect size is not something you do once in a lifetime, even if your body never changes. You will have to do some experimenting and be aware that whenever there is a basic change in fashion silhouettes, you'll probably have to check your size out all over again.

# 2
# How to build a good basic wardrobe

Think of a good basic wardrobe as a solid core of clothes that can be worn for your everyday life. If you've picked them well, these clothes will be your good friends and support you in everything you do. A little further on in this chapter we're going to tell you what we believe should be in a basic day and evening wardrobe for every woman, but first, think about your particular clothes needs. If you're like many women, you probably find yourself buying for occasions or on impulse rather than building a good workable wardrobe. We suggest you try this little experiment first, then base your clothes buying on the results.

The easiest way to assess your life in terms of clothes is to think of it as a pie with different slices for all your

## TWO DIFFERENT WARDROBE PIES

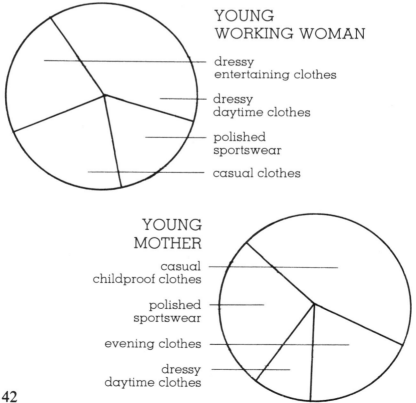

YOUNG
WORKING WOMAN

dressy
entertaining clothes

dressy
daytime clothes

polished
sportswear

casual clothes

YOUNG
MOTHER

casual
childproof clothes

polished
sportswear

evening clothes

dressy
daytime clothes

needs, the size of the slice corresponding to the importance of that area of your life. If, for example, you're a
young mother at home with two small children, a large
slice of your clothes pie will be devoted to sturdy, durable
clothes to wear during the day. If, on the other hand,
you're a working woman who entertains clients frequently, a large slice of your pie will be devoted to clothes
suitable for entertaining business associates. Here we
show you two different kinds of wardrobe "pies" repre-
senting these two women's different needs. Think of your
life and the clothes needs each part of it generates, then
draw your own pie. If the largest slice doesn't correspond
to the bulk of the clothes hanging in your closet, you have
"what to wear?" problems. Start solving them by filling
in with clothes you can wear for this part of your life.

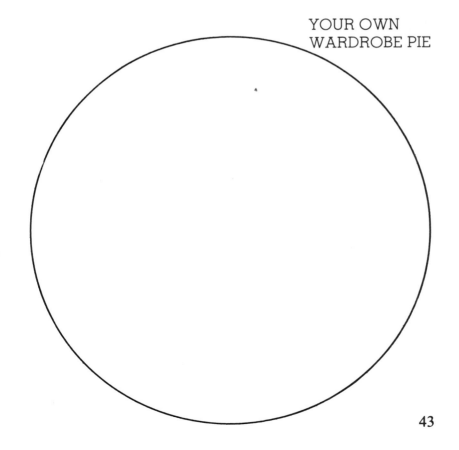

YOUR OWN
WARDROBE PIE

You will also find your wardrobe pie useful in budgeting your clothes money. The biggest, most important chunk of clothes probably deserves the largest part of your budget. Conversely, the smallest may need the least amount of money. For many women, evening clothes work out to be a small slice of the pie. Evening clothes, however, are beautiful and tempting—and often expensive—so you may find yourself overbuying here. The result can be a failed budget and clothes you may not wear enough to make them practical. Try to make your spending correspond to your real clothes needs and you'll find budgeting easier.

Once you've arrived at the clothes categories necessary for your life, the next step is the clothes themselves. We've worked out two basic wardrobes, one for day, one for evening, and we believe they will work for any woman because the choices represent enduring styles with enormous flexibility. Use these wardrobes to figure out the number of each item you yourself need, depending on how you have sliced your particular wardrobe pie.

## BASIC DAY WARDROBE

The clothes pictured on the opposite page (and in detail on the following pages) represent the backbone of a wardrobe for almost any woman. It works for a working woman or a woman who is at home raising a family, it even works for a student. The differences in these life situations is reflected in the quantity of the various items, but *all* would be represented in a well-balanced, workable wardrobe. A working woman will own more skirts, good pants, and jackets, while a woman who is at home will own more sport pants and casual clothes. The same would be true for a student.

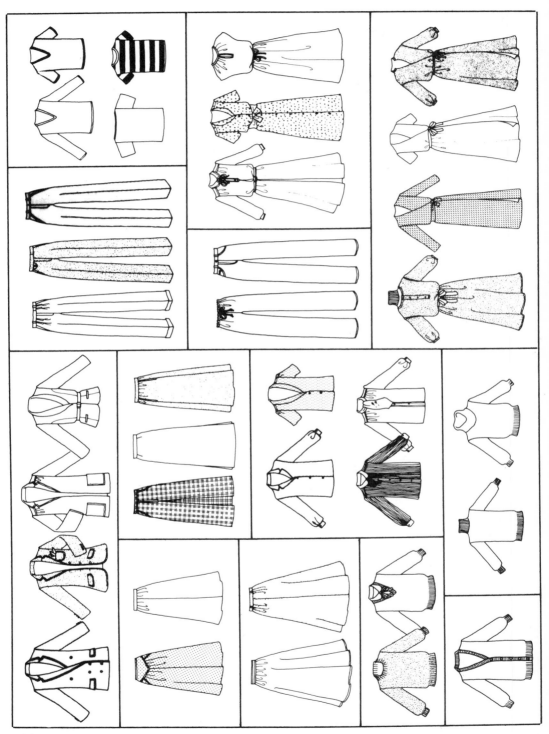

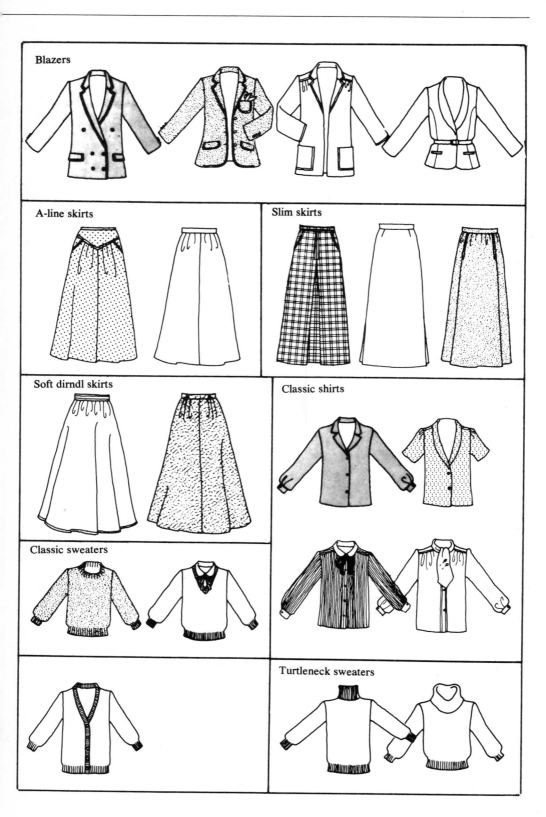

Blazers

A-line skirts

Slim skirts

Soft dirndl skirts

Classic shirts

Classic sweaters

Turtleneck sweaters

## BLAZERS

A couple of these will be the most useful items in your wardrobe. A blazer can finish a skirt, pant or dress look; it can make many looks work for day or evening.

### THE SINGLE-BREASTED BLAZER

Very classic, good over skirts, pants or dresses. Looks well open or closed. Besides putting the finish on a look, it can replace a coat in spring and fall —any blazer can.

### THE DOUBLE-BREASTED BLAZER

Classic, good over skirts or pants. Looks best buttoned, rather than open. Navy is the most basic color.

### THE SHIRT-JACKET BLAZER

More casual than the other styles, this one looks best over casual pants or skirts. It is usually worn open, rather than buttoned.

### THE BELTED BLAZER

This is a tailored choice that gives a very finished look to skirts—not the best choice for pants. Since it's belted, it's not usually worn open.

## A-LINE SKIRTS

This easy-fitting skirt is useful for almost all daytime occasions—from the office to lunch at a good restaurant. Because of its body-skimming fit, it causes few figure problems.

### YOKED A-LINE

This version fits slimly over the stomach, is softened by fullness at the hip. It works well with blouses tucked in and sweaters worn pulled down over the hip.

### CLASSIC A-LINE

Slightly softened with tucks or darts at the waist, this is the more classic of the two. It works well with blouses tucked in but is not the best choice with sweaters because tucks add too much bulk.

## SLIM SKIRTS

These skirts work well for any daytime activity. Slits or pleats give them walking ease. They are not as figure-concealing as A-line or dirndl skirts.

### CLASSIC KICK-PLEAT SKIRT

With the kick pleat in front, this skirt has all the walking ease you want and good casual style. It works equally well with sweaters or blouses.

### SLIT SKIRT

Side slits (or a rear slit) give this skirt walking ease. It works well with blouses tucked in and especially well with sweaters. If the slit is too deep, it can be too revealing for some daytime occasions.

### SIDE KICK-PLEAT SKIRT

Pleats are concealed in side seams to give walking ease. This style is more dressy than the other, looks well with blouses or sweaters.

## SOFT DIRNDL SKIRTS

These full, easy skirts are wonderful figure concealers and look well for all daytime occasions. They are good day-into-evening choices, too.

### FULL DIRNDL

This style has tucks or gathers at the waist to add fullness. It looks well with blouses tucked in. There's too much hip fullness for most sweaters.

### MODIFIED DIRNDL

Less full, this style works well with blouses or sweaters. It is the most classic of the dirndls.

## CLASSIC SHIRTS

These shirts are among the real staples of your wardrobe; you'll wear them with skirts or pants, under jackets or on their own.

### CLASSIC LONG-SLEEVE SHIRT

This is the most classic of shirts, but in a silky fabric it can go anywhere, even to an elegant restaurant.

### SHAWL-COLLARED SHIRT

This is classic but slightly more dressy than the notched collar style. It can be long or short sleeved and can go anywhere.

### SHIRT WITH CONTRASTING COLLAR AND CUFFS

This is the sportiest of the shirts. Though you can wear it with skirts, it looks especially well with casual pants.

### TIE-COLLAR SHIRT

In a silky fabric, this is the dressiest of the classic shirts. It can be worn with pants or skirts, but if you wear it with pants, don't pick the sportiest ones.

## CLASSIC SWEATERS

These V-neck or crew-neck sweaters are perfect tops for skirts or pants. Depending on the knit, they can look sporty or dressy.

### CREW-NECK SWEATER

In tweedy or cabled knits, this can look very sporty. In solid colors and fine-gauge knits, it can look dressy. Can be worn alone or over a shirt.

### V-NECK SWEATER

Cabled or tweedy styles look most sporty. Solids and fine-gauge knits look dressy. Wear it with a shirt underneath or, for a more dressy look, without. Try adding a scarf or a necklace.

⟫→

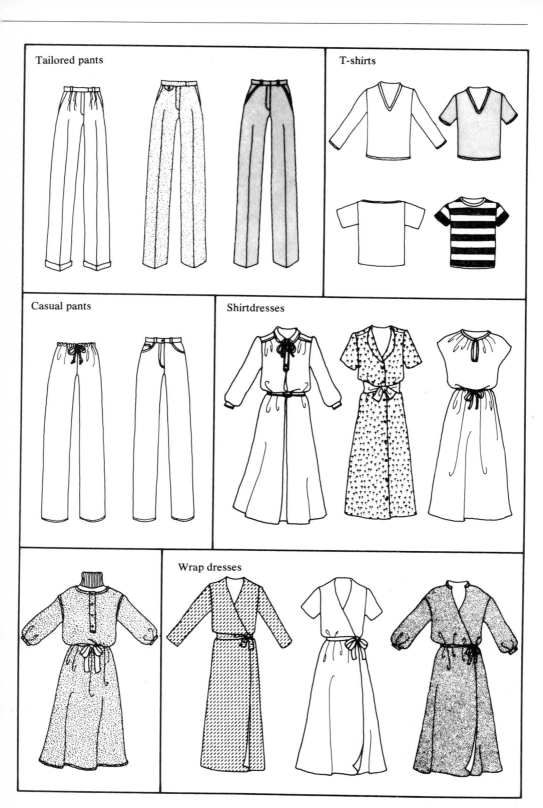

Tailored pants

T-shirts

Casual pants

Shirtdresses

Wrap dresses

CARDIGAN SWEATER
This can be worn as a jacket with a blouse under it or, for a more dressy look, alone with a scarf or necklace.

## TURTLENECK SWEATERS

### CLASSIC TURTLE
The turtleneck here fits snugly and looks more tailored. It works well with pants or skirts.

### COWL-NECK SWEATER
The cowl-neck turtle has a loose-fitting neck. It can be draped softly. It works well with pants or skirts.

## TAILORED PANTS
These straight-leg pants are tailored classically enough to go almost anywhere during the day —from the office to a community meeting to lunch out. Their effect depends greatly on how casual or dressy a top you put with them.

### PLEAT-FRONT PANTS
The front pleats of these very versatile pants give softness and help conceal large hips. Worn with a silk shirt the pants can be dressy; with a turtleneck sweater, they're casual.

### CLASSIC STRAIGHT-LEG PANTS
The most classic daytime pants, these work with blouses or sweaters. Because they fit snugly through the hip, they aren't as concealing as pleated pants.

### CLASSIC CORDUROYS
Cut like jeans but in a corduroy fabric, these pants are durable but good looking. Great with sweaters.

## T-SHIRTS
You can't have too many of these wearable favorites. Wear them with skirts or pants, for every casual occasion.

### CLASSIC V- OR CREW NECKS
Whether V-necked or crew, T-shirts are the first choice with casual pants or skirts. They are the "other half" of a pair of jeans.

## CASUAL PANTS
For casual daytime wear, you can't beat these styles. They're good at home or for outings like shopping or informal lunches.

### DRAWSTRING PANTS
These are slightly more dressy, especially if you combine them with a silky shirt. If you're wearing a sweater, try tucking it in.

### JEANS
Jeans are the "uniform" for all casual occasions when durable good looks are in order.

## SHIRTDRESSES
These are daytime wardrobe staples to wear absolutely anywhere. Wear them alone or under a jacket, to work or to church, to dinner out.

### CLASSIC SHIRTDRESS
Long-sleeved, small-collared, this is a classic, versatile dress to wear alone or under a jacket for more polish.

### SHAWL-COLLARED DRESS
Still classic, this shawl-collared style is slightly more dressy. A good choice for day into evening wear.

### SHORT-SLEEVE VERSION
Trim classic lines keep this dress in the shirtdress family. Short sleeves make it a good warm weather choice and give it day-into-evening possibilities.

### SOFT SHIRTDRESS
With a soft shoulder line and soft, full skirt, this dress is feminine, versatile and a good day-into-evening choice. It looks sporty and appealing with a turtleneck underneath. A jacket would add polish.

## WRAP DRESSES
This style wraps and ties and has a soft, feminine appeal. A wrap can go just about anywhere, has the ability to move from day-into-evening looks.

### CLASSIC WRAP
Slim, long-sleeved and classic, this dress has as much versatility as a shirtdress. A scarf or necklace dresses it up.

### SHORT-SLEEVE WRAP
Slightly more dressy, this soft-skirted style is good for all kinds of daytime wear. Can work well in the evening, too.

### SOFT WRAP
With soft sleeves and a full skirt, this is the dressiest version of the wrap dress. It works equally well day or evening. Tweedy fabrics give it a more casual feeling.

⋙→

## BASIC EVENING WARDROBE

For the majority of evening occasions, you can draw from your daytime classics, polishing them up with dressy accessories for evening. For a candlelight dinner out, for example, or for an evening at the theater, you might wear a velvet blazer, a silky shirt, and an A-line or straight skirt. You can dress up the look with bare sandals, some pretty gold or silver jewelry, or perhaps a silky scarf at your neck or around your waist. If the occasion is more dressy, you'll need to draw on your evening basics. The clothes pictured below (and in detail on the following pages) represent a good workable collection.

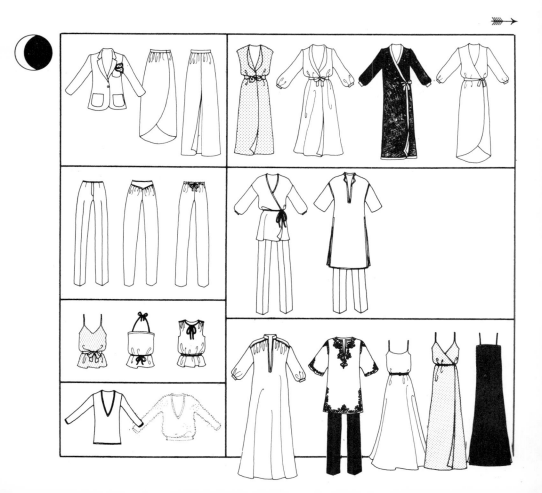

# DRESSY BLAZER

**VELVET BLAZER**
A velvet blazer is the perfect topping for dressy pants or skirt looks. It can also go over day dresses to give them evening polish.

# LONG SKIRTS

A long skirt is indispensable for entertaining at home and for occasional evenings out.

**TULIP-HEM SKIRT**
A slightly dressier long skirt that would be a good choice when you're going to a friend's home for dinner or a party. This would look well with a bare, silky top.

**CLASSIC LONG SKIRT**
A long, slim skirt is the perfect thing to wear for entertaining friends at home. A silky blouse or cowl-neck sweater would be handsome with this front-slit skirt.

# DRESSY PANTS

Any of these pants would be a good substitute for a long skirt when you're entertaining at home or going out for an evening at a friend's.

**FLY-FRONT PANTS**
The narrow leg and dressy fabric (satin, crepe, velvet) is what gives these classically cut pants a dressy look. Wear them with a silk shirt or a dressy sweater.

**YOKE-FRONT PANTS**
These slim-leg pants with a yoke and front fullness would look well with a bare top or a silky shirt. A dressy sweater would also work.

**DRAWSTRING PANTS**
In a dressy fabric and worn with a bare top or silky shirt, these pants work well for evenings at home with friends or out.

⫸→

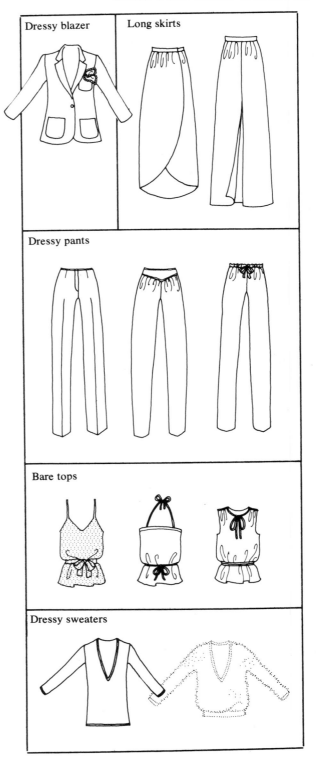

Dressy blazer

Long skirts

Dressy pants

Bare tops

Dressy sweaters

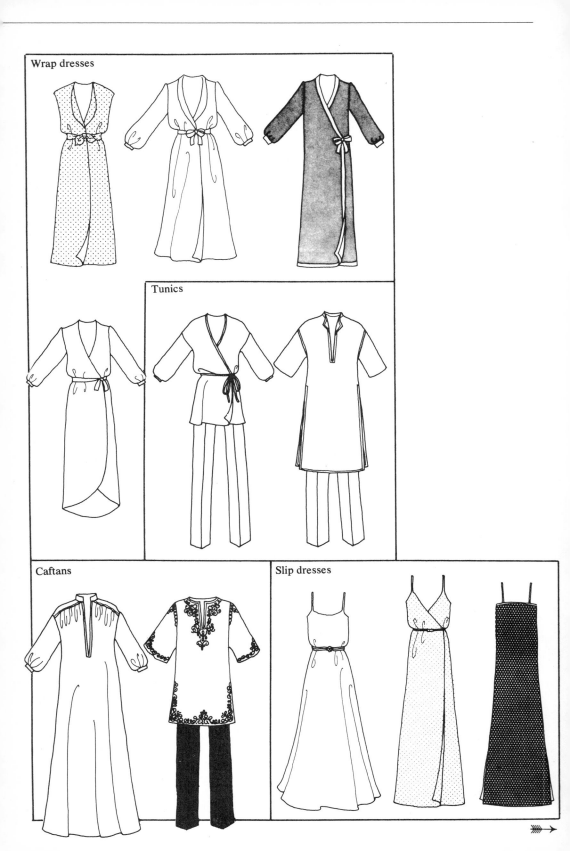

Wrap dresses

Tunics

Caftans

Slip dresses

## BARE TOPS
These are the perfect toppings for long skirts, dressy pants or for a suit in the evening.

### CAMISOLE TOPS
These bare camisole tops make skirts and pants look appealing for evening, and do wonders for even the most classic suit when worn at night.

### BARE, SLEEVELESS TOP
Not as bare and, therefore, not as dressy as a camisole, this little top looks well with velvet skirts or pants, with an evening suit or worn alone with an evening skirt.

## DRESSY SWEATERS
Imagine these in silky, lacy knits or knits flashed with metallic yarn and you have the idea.

### SKINNY SWEATER
This long, lean sweater with its deeply cut neck looks well with skinny pants in dressy fabrics. Add a glittery belt or some dressy jewelry.

### BLOUSON SWEATER
A soft sweater such as this looks best in a crochet or lacy knit or when there is a metallic gleam in the yarn. Wear it with dressy skirts or pants.

## WRAP DRESSES
These wrap and tie dresses are perfect for evening dressing. They have the ability to look "just right," not too dressed up, yet elegant and caring.

### DRESSIEST WRAP
This short-sleeved, shawl-collared wrap dress can look very dressy teamed with sandals and a metallic belt.

### FULL-SKIRTED WRAP
Soft sleeves and a full skirt create a dressy look that can go out to a restaurant, the theater or dinner at a friend's home.

### BRAID-TRIMMED WRAP
This is a good dress because it's so versatile. It's not too dressy, yet it has polish and elegance.

### TULIP-HEM WRAP
This can be quite dressy or more casual, depending on the fabric. In satin, crepe or velvet it's elegant and dressy, in wool or cotton, it's less dressy, but still can go almost anywhere except on the most formal occasions.

## TUNICS
A tunic can transform a pair of pants into a wonderful evening look. Think of these in rich fabrics such as satin or maybe even a brocade.

### SHORT TUNIC
A short tunic such as this looks well over almost any kind of slim-leg pants in a dressy fabric. Wear it at home or out.

### LONG TUNIC
In satin, silk, brocade or even velvet, this tunic worn loose over narrow-leg pants makes a wonderful at home or evening-out look.

## CAFTANS
A caftan is an evening classic. It looks marvelous at home, can go out, too.

### LONG CAFTAN
This caftan looks dressiest when lightly embroidered or when it's in a silky fabric. Because of its full shape, it's a good figure concealer.

### SHORT CAFTAN
This is perfect for at-home entertaining. It is not, however, as concealing as the long caftan if you're carrying extra weight.

## SLIP DRESSES
These dresses are always the answer when you're wondering "what to wear."

### SHORT SLIP DRESS
For a dress-up evening out, for disco dancing, for gala parties, this short slip dress is perfect.

### LONG SLIP DRESS
More elegant, more formal, this dress is versatile and always looks right when something long is called for.

Your personal wardrobe pie will guide you in deciding how many of what pieces you need, but you may find it helpful to look at the two wardrobes below first. We think they represent a minimum of clothes for a presentable wardrobe for the working woman and the young mother.

## A BASIC WORKING WOMAN WARDROBE

2 blazers—one tweedy, one velvet or in a dressy fabric that will work for day and evening
1 soft A-line skirt in seasonless fabric
1 dirndl skirt in seasonless fabric
1 slim skirt in seasonless fabric
1 pair well-tailored pants in seasonless fabric
4 classic shirts
2 pullover sweaters, either crew neck or V-neck
1 turtleneck sweater
2 shirtwaist dresses, one that can work in the evening as well as day
1 wrap dress in a soft lightweight jersey
1 pair jeans
1 pair casual sport pants
6 T-shirts
1 bare dressy top
1 long skirt

## A BASIC YOUNG MOTHER WARDROBE

2 blazers—one dressy, one sporty
1 dirndl or soft A-line skirt in seasonless fabric
3 classic shirts
2 pair of well-tailored pants
2 pullover sweaters, crew neck or V
3 turtleneck sweaters
1 shirtwaist or wrap dress in lightweight jersey
1 dressy wrap dress
4 pair jeans
2 pair sport pants
10 T-shirts
2 long skirts
1 caftan

54

You can clearly see that there is a heavy emphasis on casual clothes for the young mother since that's what she needs most of. She can get by with a minimal number of "going out" clothes because she's not likely to need many. She does, however, need something to entertain in at home—since that's a big part of her social life. The working woman needs more daytime basics to fill out her work week. She also needs to make choices that allow her to move from job to an evening look with ease. On pages 94 to 97 we show you how this can be done easily.


## ADDING THE SPARK

The clothes we've just been talking about are basics, the kind you can't do without. They are safe in terms of style. But you'll undoubtedly want more than just a collection of safe clothes. There are situations when safe dressing is exactly what you want, but there are other times when the image you want to project includes a bit of spark, perhaps even a tasteful flash. The experience of two women makes this point strikingly clear.

Claire was twenty-five, considered by her friends to be solid, conservative. What she wore to the office or on a date was predictable. Claire sometimes felt that she "blended in with the woodwork" because people didn't seem to notice her, yet she was too insecure about clothes to change and so continued to reach for the same "reliable" things in her closet. At the urging of her friend Susan, Claire let herself be "made over" for a big party both women were going to. Susan suggested Claire buy a beautiful, bare, beige jersey dress which was enormously flattering to her pale blond coloring. She sat Claire down and made up her large hazel eyes with a soft, brown eye shadow and applied more peach blusher than Claire would have dared. She picked a bright cheerful lipstick, in direct contrast to the clear gloss Claire usually wore. Claire looked smashing—and not overdone—and she was a far

55

cry from the "mouse-brown" woman everyone expected. Claire didn't meet Mr. Wonderful at the party and live happily ever after, but she did notice that people responded differently to her. People whom she hadn't met before saw only this gently sensual and very pretty woman and that's the woman they responded to. What surprised her most was what a good time she had. The experience was memorable for Claire. It made her realize that a little spark, added to her basically good but conservative image, could make people notice her and increase her pleasure in many social situations.

Kim is a thirty-year-old lawyer who usually dresses in well-cut tailored clothes and looks every inch the lawyer. She likes clothes and if she weren't a lawyer, would probably dress a lot differently. Because she'd gotten so used to reaching for the clothes with a certain severe authority when she shopped, and also because her schedule didn't give her much time to shop, she tended to wear the same kind of clothes for her private life that she wore for business. One summer weekend, Kim was invited to a friend's beach house. Kim found herself admiring the sleek white pants and bright bare tops the women wore to a Sunday brunch in her honor. Suddenly, it occured to Kim that at this moment, she wasn't Kim-the-lawyer, but just Kim-the-woman and that she, too, could wear slim white pants and a bright red top to Sunday brunch if she wished. On Monday she could go back to her more conservative workday image with no one thinking the less of her legal skills, but a lot of people thinking more of her skills at making herself an attractive woman.

There's a lot of room in most women's lives to add spark to a wardrobe. The big question is, how do you add spark without spending too much and without getting out of character? Here are some guidelines that will help:

■ Buy something in an unexpected color—unexpected for you, that is. It will add vitality. If your basic wardrobe is built around navy and gray, add a bright red silk blouse.

It will keep people from thinking you never appear in anything but basic gray or navy, yet it will go beautifully with all the good things you have in these colors.

■ Buy prints and patterns. A beautiful floral print can add a soft romantic note. A bold geometric print could add a sense of drama. Be sure one of the colors in your print or pattern will work with your basic wardrobe colors.

■ Buy something very "in." Yielding to something that's very in at the moment can be a sign that you're human and temptable, that you have a sense of fun and adventure. If you're on a tight budget, you have to exercise care here because trendy things tend to come and go pretty fast.

## WHEN IS IT A FAD AND WHEN IS IT A TREND?

A fad is something that comes and goes rather quickly and doesn't affect the mainstream of fashion. A trend affects fashion across the board, develops more slowly, and stays around longer. Investing in a trend, especially when it's fresh, can be the wisest way to add life to your basic wardrobe.

This all sounds easy enough, but how do you know whether a potential purchase represents a trend, or merely a passing fad? Here are some questions to ask yourself that will help.

Is it an item? By this we mean is it one isolated style such as a batwing sweater or stovepipe-legged pants? Isolated items that are suddenly popular tend to be fads with a short life span. A trend, on the other hand, tends to affect many items. For example, the softening up or narrowing of *all* silhouettes rather than a change in one particular one.

Is it wearable by a few or most women? If you're talking about a sudden onslaught of skintight pants or very full skirts, you're talking about something that is wearable by only a few women: those with excellent figures or perfect proportions. If you're talking about a general softening of clothes, you have something that most women can wear —and probably will like. Needless to say, there's a much better chance of the latter staying around for a while.

Now we get to the difficult question. Should you spend your hard-earned money for it? Let's assume it's a fad. Just because its life span is predictably short doesn't mean you shouldn't occasionally give a fad a whirl. What's important is that you realize it's a fad and buy with your eyes open. If it looks well on you and you will have the opportunity to wear it and can afford it—why not? One case in point: Cynthia is a twenty-five-year-old woman with a good figure. Her clothes taste runs to classic, tailored styles, but she occasionally likes to wear something really adventuresome. She found herself with invitations to three different parties during the Christmas holiday season. Cynthia decided to buy a pair of black crepe pants cut very, very narrow through the leg. She knew the style was a fad, but it was very popular at the moment, it looked well on her, and she had three places to wear the pants in the next few weeks. "Why not?" she thought, especially since she already owned tops that could change the look of the pants so that even if the same people were at two of the parties, she'd feel she looked different each time.

If a fashion change seems to be a trend, rather than a fad, your question is more likely to be *when* should you buy rather than *should* you buy. A good general rule is not to be the first to try a new look, but not the last either. If you feel the trend is harmonious with your basic sense of fashion, move in while it's fresh. The longer you wait to try it, the less mileage you'll get from your purchases and the less credit you'll get for being adventuresome.

When you feel you'd like to incorporate part of a new trend into your fashion image, consider making your first purchase something for evening or for your personal life.

Most of us feel freer about what we wear in this area than we do in a more structured business or community life. Remember how good Kim's decision to be freer in her off-hours made her feel. The best idea is to start small. Don't revamp your entire wardrobe for one new trend, no matter how much you may like it or how long-lasting it may appear to be. A closet full of romantic clothes is just as boring as a closet full of classics.

Usually one piece of clothing epitomizes a new trend. It may be the shape of a blazer or a particular kind of blouse. This is where to start. Buy what you feel is a good representation of that piece and incorporate it into your wardrobe. If this purchase works out well, you may want to add a few more things in the same mood.

Buying something new is not the only way to appear fashionably "in." You can often make subtle changes in items you already own that will make them look contemporary. For example, if belted blazers are news, you don't have to go out and buy a new blazer to have the look. You may already own a blazer whose proportions will look right when belted. Experiment in front of a mirror with belts of different widths and you'll be surprised at the results. Another example could be long, belted tunics worn with pants. Consider some of your old dresses and see if any of them could be shortened, then belted, to look interesting over pants. Try pinning up the dress first, then if you're happy with the look, cut off the dress and stitch the hem.

## COLOR HOLDS IT ALL TOGETHER

You may have most of the pieces mentioned in both the daytime and evening sections of this chapter and still legitimately complain that you don't have anything to wear. Why? Probably because you have too many separate pieces that don't work together. You put a skirt and top together and the look is unfinished or unpolished or plain doesn't work. You can solve this with color. As you've probably noticed, a great many of the clothes recommended so far have been separates. This is because they offer so much variety and so many mix-and-match possibilities. Their mood is also right for today's kind of dressing. But if your colors don't work together, you have problems. We suggest you solve this by building your basic wardrobe around two or three colors, preferably good classic colors such as beige and brown, or navy and maroon, or black, gray, and white. Your complexion and personal preference will guide you. This doesn't mean that everything in your wardrobe has to be one of these colors, but it does mean that most of the things in it will *work* with one of these colors. This way, most of the clothes hanging in your closet will mix with each other. You can add variety with highlight or accent colors that will go with your basic plan. The following chart will make this idea clear.

| BASIC COLORS | Brown/ Beige | Navy/ Maroon | Black/Gray | Navy/Red |
|---|---|---|---|---|
| ACCENT COLORS | rust shrimp coral gold tan champagne amber cognac | pale blue gray, all shades slate blue emerald green red gold | red bright green sapphire blue lilac mauve moss green white gold | bright green pale blue white wine slate blue gray, all shades |

These are not all the possibilities, but they give you a good idea of the versatility of such a system. One good plan is to buy articles such as pants and skirts in basic colors and accumulate blouses and sweaters in accent colors. Another is to keep both skirt and top in basic colors and let scarves, shoes, or jewelry be your accents.

60

You will want to add some change of pace to your basic color plan. Doing this in the evening category or in those clothes areas that belong primarily to your private life is best. It's here that you have the greatest freedom to exercise a sense of adventure and individuality. What you choose to add is important because you're making a personal statement about yourself and how you feel about the occasion. When a woman wears a bright red dress to a party, for example, she is communicating a sense of joyous expectation about the occasion. Color and its psychological and social implications are so important that we've devoted a chapter to it, starting on page 67.

## FABRIC EXTENDS WEARABILITY

More and more, clothes are becoming seasonless, and the skirt you wore in June may look equally appropriate in February. This is because of some of the wonderful new fabrics available and also to a freer, less rigid point of view about what's to be worn when. The more clothes you buy in seasonless fabrics, the more mileage you will get from your wardrobe. Depending on where you live, you may need a cluster of clothes that are only for very hot or very cold weather, but beyond that, clothes of seasonless fabrics are your best bet. The way you wear your clothes can contribute to their seasonless quality. Layering vests over shirts, sweaters over shirts, and jackets over the works gives great versatility of both look and warmth. Fabrics such as silk, silky synthetic knits, lightweight wool, wool knit, velour, lightweight gabardine, and corduroy are virtually seasonless.

Investing in seasonless clothes also solves the "between seasons" wear problem. Depending on the part of the country you live in, the transition weeks between late March and the end of May, and between September and November present "what to wear" problems. Seasonless clothes are one answer. For example, a lightweight wool or wool-blend skirt can be worn all year long. In the dead of winter you may wear it with a sweater layered over a shirt and possibly a blazer over this. In transition months, the same skirt with a shirt and blazer can work beautifully, probably both indoors and out. In full summer, you might wear the skirt with a short-sleeved blouse or dressy T-shirt. The idea of seasonless clothes and a few well-thought-out colors makes for an almost effortless kind of dressing. You put the initial effort in the shopping, from them on, it's easy.

## FABRICS CHANGE THE IMAGE

In addition to its warmth or seasonal quality, fabric can totally change the image you present. Take a blazer and skirt, for example. A velvet blazer and a wool challis skirt project a soft, feminine image. They also appear relatively dressy. Take the same shapes and think of them in deep-toned, heavy tweeds. The look suddenly becomes less soft, more authoritative or perhaps more outdoorsy, depending on the tweed. If you're aware of the subtleties fabric lends a look, you can use them to your advantage. The chart following gives you an idea of the images some fabrics tend to create. Some of the fabrics could project all three images, depending on the style and color, but in general, they do have certain associations for many people.

| IMAGE | Soft, feminine | Tailored, hard-edged |
|---|---|---|
| FABRIC | velvet<br>challis<br>silk crepe<br>soft knits<br>velours<br>satin<br>jersey<br>suede | broadcloth<br>most tweeds<br>gabardine<br>double knits<br>silk or silky<br>  twill<br>leather |

You can do some interesting things by mixing fabrics from the soft, feminine column with those in the tailored one. A young working woman, for example, might wear a velvet blazer and a gabardine skirt on a day when she is going out for dinner after work. The fabrics combine nicely and she has an image that's neither too soft nor too tailored for both occasions.

## WHAT ABOUT SPORTS CLOTHES?

What sports clothes you need depends largely on the sports or leisure activities you are involved in and how much time you have for them. Most women take sports seriously, realizing how beneficial they are to health and a general sense of well-being. Though there may be great temptation to play in whatever clothes are handy, remember that those designed for sports have a purpose. Well-designed ones make playing easier because they allow maximum freedom of movement and ease. You don't want to feel constricted or uncomfortable in action.

Before you buy anything meant for serious sports activity, try it on, move about in it to be sure it fits well and doesn't bind. Shop in stores specializing in sports clothes. You'll usually find a better selection at good prices.

If you need another reason to invest in good sports clothes, remember that you are likely to be highly visible on public courts. A game of tennis or squash with business colleagues is also becoming as popular with women, before or after work, as it is with men. In this case, your business image overlaps a personal one and how you look is important.

## HOW TO CHOOSE YOUR ACCESSORIES

Don't overlook the importance of accessories. They can make the difference between a day or an evening look, a casual or more polished one. They can make a look summery or wintery, just right or just off. The sketches below include a basic group every woman should aim for. You can see right away that a pair of boots, for example, can create a winter feeling while a pair of bare sandals can give the same outfit either a more dressy look or a warm-

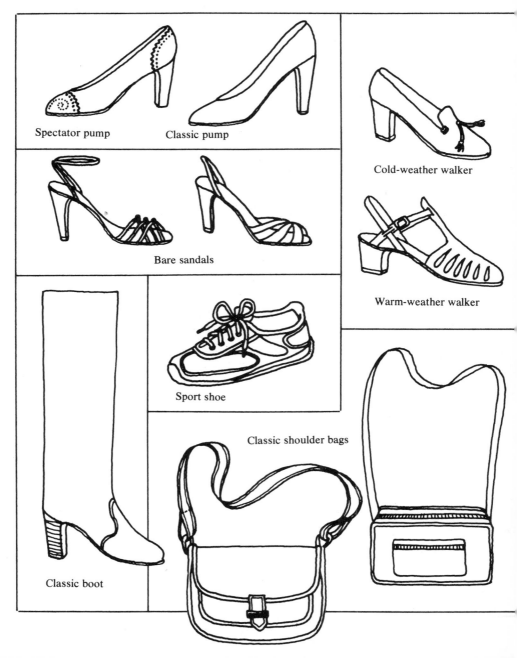

Spectator pump     Classic pump

Bare sandals

Cold-weather walker

Warm-weather walker

Sport shoe

Classic shoulder bags

Classic boot

weather feeling. Walking shoes can give a sporty look to a blazer, shirt, and skirt, while sandals would dress this outfit up. A wrap dress in a knit can go summer or winter with a change of shoes and jewelry. Sandals and a wooden bead necklace for summer could replace the gold chains and pumps of winter.

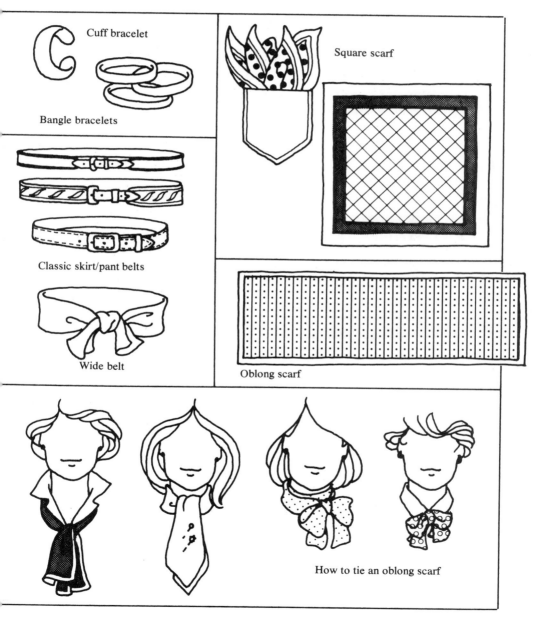

Cuff bracelet

Bangle bracelets

Classic skirt/pant belts

Wide belt

Square scarf

Oblong scarf

How to tie an oblong scarf

## TIPS FOR YOUNG MOTHERS

Probably no one puts clothes to a greater test than a young mother keeping up with a small child. What you need are clothes that wash well, stand up to spills, and are good-looking, too. Many young women rely on jeans and jean skirts because they are sturdy and comfortable, but you don't want to be like the young mother who complained that she felt her jeans were a permanent extension of her body! To relieve the monotony, consider skirts and pants in blends of cotton and polyester in twill weaves and soil-resistant colors such as khaki, gray, forest green or navy. A variety of T-shirts and man-tailored shirts in bright colors will pick up the pants or skirts. T-shirts in the medium price range are worth the money. They wash better and keep their shape longer. A blazer jacket in a heavy tweedy fabric will look well over any of these clothes when you're outdoors in mild weather. For colder days, a good-looking parka or poncho is useful.

If you have just made the transition from working woman to mother, you will find it invaluable to accumulate some of these sturdy, but good-looking clothes quickly. Many young women tell us that the temptation to stay in a robe in the morning while you do chores that are likely to soil clothes is overwhelming, but may contribute, usually unconsciously, to a sense of depression. Keeping a schedule you set for yourself and that involves putting on makeup and good-looking, comfortable clothes is worth the effort. Changing at the end of the day, usually just before dinner is another spirit lifter. With the great variety of casual but handsome pants around now—gathered and wrapped waists, pleats, drawstrings—you can enjoy the lift and variety they give. Most of them go easily into a washing machine and require little or no pressing. A caftan in a washable fabric is another pretty dinner-hour idea.

66

# 3
# Color:
# How you can make its psychological implications work for you

In the last chapter we talked about color and how sticking to a few basic ones can make shopping easier and can simplify putting different looks together. We also pointed out that wearing monotones or at least shades of one color can help elongate a short body and how certain deep colors can give heavy bodies a slimmer appearance. Color can do much more than this. It can make people feel warm or cool toward you; it can help you assume a more aggressive or persuasive attitude, or, conversely, a more passive one. It can make you noticeable or make you fade into the background. In this chapter, we're going to talk about the effects color has on your emotions and on those of the people around you.

## COLOR RESPONSES ARE LEARNED

Psychologists say that color means different things to different people and the whole field of color aesthetics is a very controversial one. Most psychologists do agree, however, that color aesthetics are learned and that they are basically cultural. In other words, children don't respond to oranges and yellows as "warm" colors or blue and white as "cool" colors as much as adults do because they haven't *learned* to make this association yet. Western cultures often don't share the same set of color aesthetics as Eastern cultures. But since we are primarily concerned with the responses we get from other adults in

68

our own culture, it seems appropriate enough to make certain associations about color and emotion.

Color goes to your head: it can stimulate, excite, depress, annoy, soothe and generally affect your state of mind directly. Psychologists have actually been able to show in the laboratory that warm colors such as red, yellow, or orange can raise blood pressure or temperature and stimulate appetite. Red can step up heartbeat, blue can slow it down. We obviously associate certain emotional states with color—think of "seeing red" when you're angry or "feeling blue" when you're depressed.

## PLEASURE AND AROUSAL COLORS

One of the most interesting ideas about color, in terms of its potential for dressing, comes from Albert Mehrabian, an environmental designer who is associated with the University of California at Los Angeles. He has found that most of us respond emotionally to a range of colors which he has divided into pleasure colors and arousal colors. Pleasure colors are shades of blue, green, purple, red, and yellow—listed from most to least pleasurable. Arousal colors, those stimulating an emotional reaction either positive or negative, are shades of red, orange, yellow, violet, blue, and green—again listed from most to least arousing. There are three components of color that are important in affecting your reaction: hue, saturation, and brightness. The hue of a color simply means its wavelength on a light spectrum. It's what gives a color its color. A color's saturation is its depth or concentration. Brightness is a color's ability to reflect light. Saturation has a direct relationship to arousal. As you increase the saturation of a color, you increase its arousal qualities. For example, a pale pastel orange would have fewer arousal qualities than a deep, concentrated orange. As you increase the brightness of a color, you also increase

69

its arousal qualities. You might keep the following tips in mind when you're picking clothing colors for an important occasion:

■ If you want to stimulate someone's emotions, wear high-pleasure and high-arousal colors. Red, violet or purple, for example.
■ To relax and calm, wear high-pleasure but low-arousal colors, such as blue or green.
■ To induce anxiety or provoke fear, wear low-pleasure and high-arousal colors, such as yellow or red.
■ To bore, wear low-pleasure and low-arousal colors, such as green or yellow.
■ A high-arousal color with high saturation and low brightness is most likely to make your presence dramatically felt. A deep, concentrated red would be a good example.

Needless to say, these are not foolproof tips, both because not everyone responds alike to a given color and because there is often a fine line between whether a color is pleasing or arousing and to what degree. To make color work for, not against you, especially when the situation is an important one, say a job interview, a meeting with an important client, a public talk, it's worth your while to do some thinking about the colors you wear. The idea worked for one woman.

Helen is a young lawyer who was going to present her first case in court before a judge and jury. She was understandably nervous and determined to make a good impression. She had two different outfits she was considering wearing for the trial: one, a conservative gray suit with a blazer jacket and a classic pleated skirt; the other, a deep red jersey wrap dress. Helen's husband felt the gray suit was most appropriate for the courtroom; it was conservative and the color wouldn't stand out, in fact, it would probably be repeated in the color of other

70

male lawyer's suits. Helen considered her husband's opinion, but in the end she decided to wear the red dress. She is a competent lawyer and she had done all her homework so she presented her case convincingly. But what Helen recalls now is the way most of the jury's eyes followed her as she moved dramatically around the courtroom giving her final summation of the case. They couldn't seem to take their eyes from her and she was never sure how much this might have had to do with her red dress.

No one would say that Helen won her case because she wore a red dress, but it indeed may have made the job of winning easier by making what she said and the way she said it more dramatic.

Colors have negative as well as positive effects and you can often use these negative effects to your own advantage. Low-pleasure and high-arousal colors have been shown to provoke fear and anxiety. Imagine yourself in the position of Susan, a young woman who lives in an apartment building in a large metropolitan area. There have been two robberies in the building lately, and fearful that hers might be the next apartment burglarized, Susan organized a tenants' meeting in the lobby of her building. Susan's aim was to interest everyone in persuading the landlord to install a TV security system in the building. The lobby of Susan's building is painted a soft French blue, a high-pleasure color. Susan happened to be wearing a peacock-blue dress, again a high-pleasure color. Tenants sitting in the peaceful, pleasant blue lobby didn't feel much anxiety and didn't like the idea of unattractive TV cameras interrupting the serenity of the building entrance. They had a doorman, they said, and the two robberies were probably the result of carelessness in the burglarized apartments. Would the outcome of the meeting have been different if Susan had chosen the other public room in the building, a meeting room in the basement decorated in yellow, a low-pleasure, relatively high-arousal color more likely to set the scene for tension that a soft, restful blue?

71

Would it have helped if Susan had chosen a low-pleasure, high-arousal color to wear? No one can say for sure, but many executives, working from Mehrabian color ideas, have decorated their offices with low-pleasure, high-arousal colors to reinforce their own aura of authority. Theatrical set designers, TV designers, and home decorators all take advantage of color's ability to stimulate people emotionally. Women have an edge here because they can dress in many more colors than men do and use color to help reinforce certain moods.

## COLOR ASSOCIATIONS

We started this chapter by saying that the field of color aesthetics is a controversial one. The pleasure and arousal color theory we have just been talking about, though appealing, is only *one* theory. There are others. The chart that follows shows you the findings of two well-known color researchers, Dr. Max Lüscher and Faber Birren. You might like to check out your favorite colors and see what associations people have reported about them.

| COLOR | PLEASANT ASSOCIATIONS | UNPLEASANT ASSOCIATIONS |
|---|---|---|
| Red | exciting, stimulating, loving, powerful, strong, warm, human | agressive, disturbing, vulgar, bloody, defiant |
| Orange | friendly, jovial, incandescent, social | intrusive, gaudy, blustering |
| Yellow | sunny, cheerful, optimistic, expansive, radiant | glaring, imperious, bilious, eccentric |
| Green | tranquil, quiet, consoling, comforting, natural | commonplace, tiresome |
| Blue | calm, comfortable, secure | depressing, melancholy, lonely, cold |
| Violet | regal, exclusive, dignified | conceited, funereal, esoteric, pompous |
| Brown | dependable, steady, reliable | clumsy, boring, dour, stingy, obstinate |
| Pink | dainty, sweet, gentle, tender | effete, effeminate, saccharine |
| White | innocent, hopeful, celestial, spiritual | sterile, glaring, unemotional, bleak |
| Gray | secure, peaceful, protective, safe | dreary, tedious, passive, negative, colorless |
| Black | sophisticated | deathly, ominous, empty, fatal |

## COLOR PERSONALITIES

It is true that certain assumptions are made about people who like particular colors. Researcher Faber Birren has put together some of the more common associations of people and colors. Reading them has all the fun and suspense of having your fortune told. Here are a few of the most common associations:

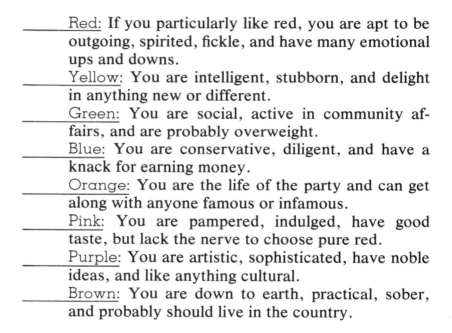

    <u>Red</u>: If you particularly like red, you are apt to be outgoing, spirited, fickle, and have many emotional ups and downs.

    <u>Yellow</u>: You are intelligent, stubborn, and delight in anything new or different.

    <u>Green</u>: You are social, active in community affairs, and are probably overweight.

    <u>Blue</u>: You are conservative, diligent, and have a knack for earning money.

    <u>Orange</u>: You are the life of the party and can get along with anyone famous or infamous.

    <u>Pink</u>: You are pampered, indulged, have good taste, but lack the nerve to choose pure red.

    <u>Purple</u>: You are artistic, sophisticated, have noble ideas, and like anything cultural.

    <u>Brown</u>: You are down to earth, practical, sober, and probably should live in the country.

## HOW DO YOU INTERPRET COLOR THEORIES

As interesting as all these color theories are, they can be confusing. Which, if any, do you pay attention to? All the theories mentioned here have been worked out by respected researchers and represent some of the most commonly held ideas. We're not recommending that you decide what mood you want to create each day and then pick a color that will do it. Color can be most useful to you in a fashion sense if you use it as we suggested in the last chapter, that is, to hold your wardrobe together by selecting a couple of good basic colors as a backbone, then building looks around these. In addition to this, however, there are those times when the impression you want to create is especially important. These are the times when it is worthwhile to make use of the power some colors seem to have to stir certain predictable emotional responses. You will notice that some colors seem to have similar emotional connotations in most of the color theories. Purple, for example, is considered to be regal and sophisticated by many researchers. Red is considered a strong, highly emotional color. Pick out the similarities in the color theories and remember that these similarities probably represent the strongest cases for assuming that color will help precipitate a particular emotional response.

## DO YOU REINFORCE YOUR OWN EMOTIONS WITH COLOR?

If color is able to affect the moods and emotions of others, it follows that it affects yours, too—perhaps more subtly than you imagine. Why, on some days when you're feeling blue and depressed, do you reach for the dreariest dress in your closet? Why do you tend to pick something bright and cheerful when you're feeling good? In doing these things, you're probably using color to reinforce your own moods which can be a self-destructive process. Consider the experiences of these two women.

Denise is an attractive, generally cheerful woman who is a first-rate public relations writer. She had an opportunity to interview for a job with a major public relations firm. The job represented a step up in both salary and prestige. The day before the interview, when Denise opened her mailbox, she found a rejection slip from a magazine for a short manuscript she had recently submitted. The rejection disappointed and upset her. When she dressed for her interview the next morning, she unconsciously chose one of the dreariest dresses she owned. It was dark gray, high-necked and since she was feeling blah, she didn't take the time to liven it up with a colorful scarf or some jewelry. When she checked herself in the mirror before leaving home, her self-esteem slipped another notch because she felt she looked so drab. She later felt her performance at the interview was as colorless as she looked. She got the job, but several months after she started working, her boss, who had interviewed her, confided that she almost didn't hire her because her manner was so low-key and she looked so mousy and drab that her boss wondered if Denise would fit the image of the firm. Her credentials were good and her writing was first-class so her boss wisely chalked off her appearance to nerves or a bad day—but it was a close call.

Sarah and Hank were going to celebrate their first wedding anniversary with a candlelight dinner at a luxurious restaurant. She and Hank had a fight over the phone that morning and it took the edge off the occasion for Sarah and made her feel depressed. As she dressed for dinner that evening, she just didn't feel like putting on the pretty, yellow chiffon print she had originally planned to wear. Instead, she wore a black crepe dress she had never particularly liked. The somber mood of the dress seemed to set the key for the evening, and all in all, it was not an evening she cared to remember.

What both Sarah and Denise did was use color to reinforce a negative mood. They felt blue and depressed and they chose colors that intensified the mood rather than something that might have helped brighten their spirits. If Denise had made the effort to wear something she particularly liked and felt good in, the whole tone of her interview well might have been more upbeat. If Sarah had worn her chiffon dress, it might have made her feel pretty and gay and encouraged her to act that way.

Many women say that they know what kind of a day

they're going to have when they pick a particular dress or outfit in the morning. "When I wear this dress," says one woman, "I always feel good and attractive and it makes me feel better no matter what happens during the day." Conversely, another woman reports, "I can't explain it, but whenever I wear this dress I have a lousy day. I feel unattractive and I'm grumpy." Clothes, especially their color, obviously affect our moods. Choosing a dress in a color (and of course a style) you like can help you feel confident and attractive. If you have had an unpleasant emotional experience or you're going into a particularly tense situation, wear something you like. It will make you feel good about yourself and help offset some of the tensions or depressed feelings you may have.

## HOW MUCH COLOR CAN YOU HANDLE?

Depending on the occasion, this can be an important question. Let's say you decide to go all out for the party and you wear a bright red, very close-fitting dress. You may look sensational, but do you *feel* comfortable? This is not the kind of color or style that will allow you to fade into the crowd and go unnoticed. If you would feel more relaxed mixing with, rather than standing out from the crowd, wear something quieter.

Color can make you the focus of attention in business as well as social situations. If you're participating in a panel discussion, for example, and you haven't had the time to do as much boning up on the subject as you'd like, you'd do best choosing a neutral color rather than red or purple. Dressed in the bright color, you stand out more and what you say is more likely to be remembered. You're also more likely to have questions directed to you in a question and answer session.

# 4
# What to wear when

A friend once confessed that she gets terrible nervous butterflies in her stomach every time she goes to a party. "When I was thirteen," she said, "I was invited to my first 'grown-up' party. I spent hours bathing, washing my hair, and putting on my first pink blush of lip color, and finally stepping into the white party dress my mother bought for me. I could hardly wait to get to the party, but once there, I was horrified. There I stood, in my short white dress with shiny white patent leather shoes, looking out at a room full of my contemporaries *all* in long 'sophisticated' dresses."

We all have at least one similar memory that years later still makes us cringe with embarrassment. That memory is so profound it often impels us "to look like everyone at the party" for the rest of our lives. The ideas in this chapter are not meant to tell you precisely what to wear when or to give you the impression that there is only one right choice. They *are* intended to give you some reliable clothes options which will work in many different situations and leave you feeling relaxed and ready to get on with the business at hand.

Everytime you step outside your door, you've made a decision about what you're wearing. Often this is an important decision because the success of your plans may be crucially affected by it. To see just how tricky it can all be, try your hand at the quiz below.

# WHAT WOULD <u>YOU</u> WEAR?

1. *You have a job interview for a spot that represents a move upward in your career. Would you wear:*

    (a) a silk shirt and skirt
    (b) a gabardine pantsuit
    (c) a gabardine skirt suit?

2. *You are attending the meeting of your local PTA with your husband. Would you wear:*

    (a) a turtleneck sweater and wool pants
    (b) a wrap jersey dress
    (c) a wool suit?

3. *You and a date are going to the theater with another couple. Would you wear:*

    (a) a long skirt and silk blouse
    (b) a dressy jersey outfit
    (c) a gabardine suit?

4. *You and your husband are going to a friend's house for dinner. Would you wear:*

    (a) a skirt and silk shirt
    (b) a sweater and pants
    (c) a long skirt and dressy top?

5. *You are meeting your future mother-in-law for lunch in town. Would you wear:*

    (a) a tailored wool suit
    (b) a dressy silk blouse and skirt
    (c) a sweater and wool pants?

6. *You are going to a country inn for lunch on a Sunday with your beau. Would you wear:*

    (a) a wrap jersey dress
    (b) a tailored wool suit
    (c) a turtleneck and wool pants?

## Scoring

If you chose option (a), the silk shirt and skirt, you were right. If you chose option (b), the gabardine pantsuit, you were right, too. If you chose (c) the gabardine skirt suit, you were also right. In fact, *all* the options in *all* the questions are right. They could almost all be wrong, too, depending on the situation and what's appropriate for it. This points out clearly that there is no *one* right answer to most clothes questions. *Appropriate* is the key word here. Deciding what is appropriate to wear in any given circumstance involves assessing many things about that situation: the time of day, how formal you consider it, what the others present will be wearing and probably most important of all, what impression you want to create. Your decision involves judgment and it takes experience to develop the kind of judgment that won't let you down, no matter where you're going. Though no one can tell you unfailingly what will be right, it is possible to develop a technique that will help you assess the essentials of important clothes decisions so that you come out a winner.

## DEVELOPING AN EYE

Learning to be a good observer is crucial to making successful clothes choices. You should observe what people whose value system is important to you consider appropriate dress in varous situations. Again, appropriate is the all-important word, it's not a question of right or wrong. The girl in the white party dress looked "right" to her mother, but to her peers, she looked like a child at a grown-up party. Consequently she felt acutely embarrassed. You can save yourself similar embarrassment and anxiety if you become a good observer, storing away facts about what you observe so that you can use them later.

For example, when you go to the theater or a concert on a weekday evening, you might notice that most people are dressed casually in skirts and blouses or casual dresses. There are only a few women wearing long skirts or dressy cocktail dresses. From your observations, you can conclude that you will be appropriately dressed if you pick casual clothes for this kind of event any time in the future. You may also observe that on a Saturday evening you see many more long skirts and really dressy looks. This is probably because most people tend to feel more festive on the weekend and they also are more likely to combine the theater with a restaurant dinner or a party. Some people call this kind of observation "people watching" and it can be a useful as well as an amusing pastime.

## ASKING THE RIGHT QUESTIONS

When you're in doubt about what to wear, ask questions, as many as you can. Consider this example: you're invited to a party on a weekend evening. The invitation is by telephone so you have the perfect opportunity to ask your hostess what kind of party it is, whether it's a casual get-together or a more formal one. Your questions can be subtle and not off-putting, but they can provide you with the information you need. Here are some helpful questions to ask yourself or someone else.

Q. *Is it a large or small gathering?*

A. Large parties, gatherings, etc. tend to be more formal and reserved (except cocktail parties) than small ones, and people usually dress accordingly.

Q. *How formal is it?*

A. The more formal and elegant the setting (restaurant, reception hall, etc.) the more formal and "dressed up" people tend to get.

83

Q. *Is it a day or evening occasion?*

A. Daytime meetings, dates, and restaurant outings are usually more casual than those in the evening.

Q. *Is it in the city or the suburbs?*

A. City meetings, dates, events are usually more "dressy" than those in the country or suburbs.

Q. *Is it on a weekend or a weekday?*

A. Weekend festivities are likely to be more dressy than those in midweek.

Q. *If I have no clues at all, in which direction should I lean?*

A. When in doubt about how to dress, you'll usually feel more comfortable if you err on the conservative side. An elegant casual look will seem more appropriate in a dressy setting than looking "all dressed up" when everyone else is casual.

Q. *Long dress or short?*

A. When in doubt about wearing a long dress or short one, opt for the short. You'll undoubtedly have company in your choice whereas you may not if you pick the long one.

Q. *How can I make a big impression?*

A. If you want to make a strong impression and stand out from the crowd, wear something that's an "in" fashion. Look to a reliable fashion magazine for good choices.

## USEFUL CLOTHES CHOICES

The best clothes choices are versatile enough to go many places. Below, we give you some good choices for a few of the most common social situations.

Restaurants: If you're lunching at a good restaurant in a city environment, any kind of wrap jersey dress, a shirtwaist dress, a suit, a silky shirt and skirt, a blazer, shirt, and skirt will do beautifully. A well-put-together skirt and sweater look would also work. If you go this casually, wear a handsome silk scarf and a piece of jewelry to "dress up" your sweater look. A pair of well-cut pants and a silky shirt could also work—unless it's a business lunch. You would want to look more polished in this situation and should probably choose a suit, a blazer, shirt and skirt combination, or a dress and blazer jacket.

If your restaurant date is for dinner, most of the lunch options would still work, but you would want to pick slightly dressier versions of these looks. The shirt should be a soft blouse of some kind, the wrap dress might be in a dressier fabric, say a silky knit. You might wear a velvet blazer rather than a wool one. A satin blazer and a skirt or dressy tapered-leg pants would be a handsome look for a dressy dinner.

Little dates: If your date is a movie and a bite to eat, you can consider it pretty casual and pick a shirt and skirt or pants, a dress and blazer, maybe a corduroy blazer, or a sweater and skirt. Any of these put-togethers would also work for a casual dinner in an informal restaurant, a lecture, or a drive in the country.

Big dates: This really depends on where you're going, but keep in mind that if you consider it a "big" date, it's probably because you want to impress your date and look special. Understated but elegant is a good look to aim for. If the occasion is formal, say a dance, a dinner party in someone's home, or a cocktail party, consider a midcalf or ankle-length slip dress, one with a camisole or slip top and shoestring straps, or a very dressy blouse and an ankle-length skirt. Subtle details such as a deep slit in a skirt or a deeply V'ed neckline on a shirt can be construed as dressy, yet keep you from looking overdressed in situations where you're not quite sure how dressed up you're expected to be. A few dressy accessories like a pair of glittery earrings or bracelets can do the same job.

Events: This can be anything from a PTA meeting to the local meeting of the League of Women Voters. Dressing conservatively is the wisest choice. A suit, a blazer jacket, skirt, and shirt, a jersey dress would all be good choices. Add some polish with a good-looking scarf or the subtle gleam of a piece of gold jewelry, but don't overdo it.

## THE WORKING WOMAN

In this country today, 50.4 percent of all working age women work; in fact, women comprise 41.2 percent of the country's total work force. The number of working women is rising so rapidly it's difficult to keep pace with the figures. The most important aspect of this phenomenon is that a large percentage of these women are not just working, they are planning a career and for them, what to wear is part of the plan.

### The Job Interview

Before any job, there's the job interview, a face-to-face confrontation that probably makes you feel as vulnerable as you're ever going to feel. This is the one time when the whole purpose of you're being present is to be evaluated. It is a tension-producing situation if there ever was one, and if you don't feel relaxed about the way you look, it will add to your anxiety. Looking right can make a considerable difference in how you are perceived, as you will see from the survey recently conducted by *Glamour*. We sent to personnel directors all across the country photographs of one woman dressed five different ways. (One woman so that we could rule out the possibility of the interviewer responding to the physical characteristics of a particular woman rather than to what she was wearing.) These personnel directors represented all kinds of firms, from advertising agencies to insurance companies and in each case, we asked the people making the evaluations to assume that the interviewee was applying for a management training job and that she was well qualified. You see photographs of the five looks on pages 89 to 91. We expected that there might be a major difference in the attitude of a conservative firm, such as an insurance company or a stock brokerage, as compared to a more liberal organization, such as an advertising agency. There wasn't. Opinion was consistent, leading us to believe that on a management trainee level, most firms are looking for much the same kind of image.

Overwhelmingly, the personnel directors responded negatively to the woman dressed in the rigidly tailored pantsuit, look 4. Almost all commented on her severe look, not just the suit itself, but the severity of her hairstyle and minimal makeup as well. We heard comments such as these: "This look projects too much inflexibility," "She has totally denied her femininity," "I do not feel that women need to appear masculine in order to be successful in a male-dominated business world." We thought it significant that some of the directors completely ignored this candidate and did not even mention her in their responses.

The overwhelming winner in this survey was number 1, a conservative but definitely feminine look. About this look, we heard comments like these: "She appears smart, serious, and able to handle any event of a business day." "I would offer the job to this woman because, on the basis of visual impact, the total look results in a serious, self-assured image. She does not deny her femininity."

Surprisingly, the runner-up was look number 5, a very soft, feminine look. About this woman, we heard these comments: "A sharp, sleek impression, compatible with a changing fashion trend for the contemporary business-woman. "A bit more avant-garde than the woman in photograph 1, but obviously 'smart' looking."

Most personnel directors felt look number 3 was a perfectly good look, but somehow unfinished. What seemed to be missing here was some sort of jacket. "The overall impression is softer [than look 4] more feminine, but still tailored and businesslike. If she had a matching jacket, she would have been first choice."

We were not surprised by the reaction to look number 2. Almost everyone felt that the combination of hairstyle and accessory choice was too "trendy" to be taken seriously—except in fields where this kind of look is appropriate such as a fashion or advertising business or the entertainment industry. One quote sums up the reaction: "This outfit is not suitable for a management trainee. Her scarf is inappropriate, sweater too baggy, her hair looks unkempt, and she is wearing too much makeup."

From this survey, we concluded that clothes that somehow get across the feeling of polish, of a professionally competent image, that are serious but not rigid are ideal choices for a job interview. There is no doubt that now and probably for a long time to come, the surest choice is some kind of suit look or a dress and jacket. It speaks with unmistakable authority. Keep what you put with it in the same classic mood—handbag, shoes, even hair and makeup, and you won't go wrong. Once you've put yourself together appropriately, you're free to give your undivided attention to the other details of the interview—such as selling your abilities and skills.

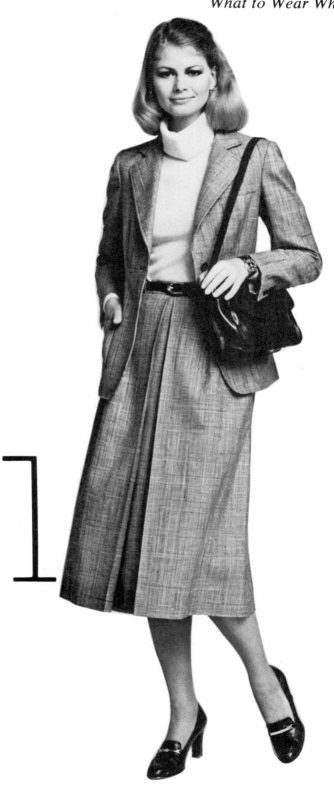

1

2 3

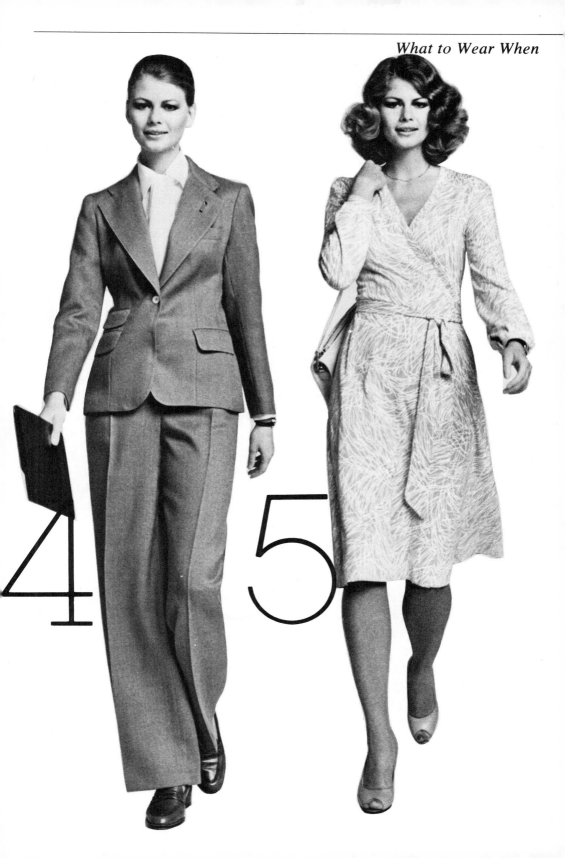

4  5

A job interview is like a first date. It gives you a first impression of another person, tells you whether you want to continue the relationship, but it doesn't really tell you much about how the day-to-day living will be—and that, after all, is what a job is all about. After you've landed the job, the most important part of your strategy begins. Your looks are as crucial to getting ahead as they were to getting the job in the first place.

If you want to get ahead, dress as if you're already there. Put another way, pick the job you aspire to and dress as if you have that job. Some women have found it useful to pattern themselves after the successful women in their firm. If these women have made it, they theorize, looking the way they do must have helped. It certainly didn't hurt. We don't recommend you actually pattern yourself on anyone. You have to be yourself, to feel comfortable and express your own uniqueness. It is wise, however, to be aware of the kinds of clothes that are worn in your company, especially by the successful people. Unless you have something very special to offer, you're going to have to fit into that corporate picture. If you find this picture too restrictive, it could well be that the corporation or field itself will restrict you too much to develop your special talents.

If there are no women authority figures in your company you can translate the men's dress into something you can relate to. (You may also want to ask yourself if you have valid reasons for feeling that you will succeed in rising in authority where other women have not.) If yours is an office where men never remove their jackets, if white or very conservative shirts and ties are all you see, you can assume you will be expected to maintain a rather conservative image, too.

Even in relatively conservative companies, you will see "successful" workers dressed casually. One woman executive we know said, "I let my assistant come in dressed in jeans because she's very good and I value her, but I wouldn't promote her to a more visible job. Our clients would never stand for it.'' When asked why she wouldn't just promote the woman and ask her to dress differently, the executive replied, ''If I have to tell her something like that, she's not going to work out in the long run.'' Dressing ''up the ladder'' in a job says more about you than you may be aware of. It communicates that you see yourself as someone who's going to get ahead and that subtle message can help considerably in your plan to get there. Don't underestimate its value.

## Looks That Should Never Make It to the Office

No matter what kind of work situation you're in, there are some things that should never appear, if you want to be considered a serious contender for the next job up.

- See-through clothing
- Obviously tight or sexy clothes
- Bare midriffs
- Very bare sundresses (unless circumstances are unusual: it's 95° and the air conditioning breaks down.)
- Rumpled, generally mussed-up clothes
- Clothes so trendy they distract everyone in sight
- Anything that looks as though it belongs in a disco or nightclub.

## The Problem of the After-Office Date

One of the most universal "what to wear" problems of working women is the after-the-office date when you must go directly from work into a situation that calls for a dressier look. There are some very good solutions that don't require you to carry a suitcase to the office or to look overdressed all day.

Most women keep a small cosmetic kit in their offices so they can freshen makeup before going out. No more trouble and equally as useful is an extra pair of shoes, preferably a go-with-everything pair of high-heeled sandals. They are invaluable in dressing up an ordinary look. An "emergency" pin or necklace that adds a dressy touch is also useful to have stowed away in a drawer.

When you know ahead of time that you're going out in the evening, plan ahead. A wrap jersey dress, for example, would work well. For office wear you might have a pretty scarf at the neck; when you go out, you can remove the scarf to show off bare skin. A shirtwaist dress or anything that buttons up the front can look more dressy unbuttoned a bit to show more skin. A suit, especially one with a soft jacket, perhaps with a shawl collar, is a great idea. You can wear the suit with a shirt and no jacket during the workday. When it's time to go out, take off the shirt, put on the soft jacket, belting it or buttoning it so that is shows some skin at the neck and looks soft and attractive. The sketches on pages 95 to 97 will give you some ideas. A velvet blazer could be made to work the same way. Try it buttoned with no shirt and consider adding a dressy belt of some kind. You could also easily carry an extra dressier shirt to exchange for the one you've worn all day. If you normally carry a big handbag, you might consider making do with something smaller and more dressy on a day you know you're going out directly from the office.

If your hair is long enough to put up or to arrange in a more festive style, change it before you leave the office.

94

Take advantage of the boost some fragrance can give you, too. If you're not in the habit of wearing it during working hours, do keep some in your desk so that you can use it when you go out.

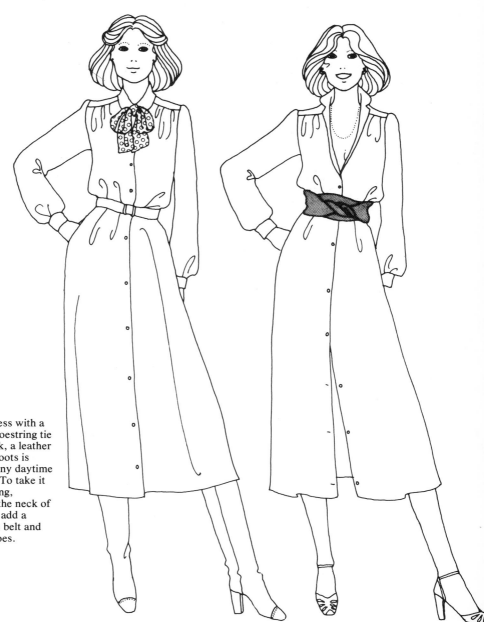

A shirt dress with a narrow shoestring tie at the neck, a leather belt and boots is great for any daytime occasion. To take it into evening, unbutton the neck of the dress, add a narrow tie belt and dressy shoes.

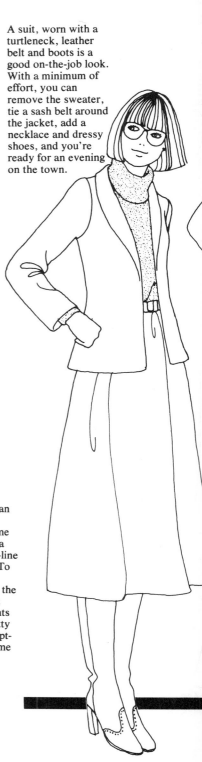

A suit, worn with a turtleneck, leather belt and boots is a good on-the-job look. With a minimum of effort, you can remove the sweater, tie a sash belt around the jacket, add a necklace and dressy shoes, and you're ready for an evening on the town.

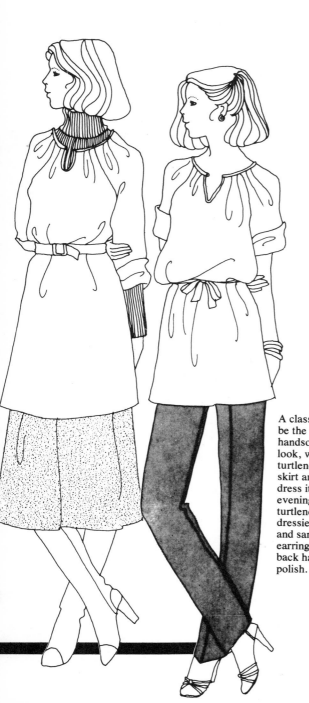

A classic tunic can be the basis of a handsome daytime look, worn with a turtleneck, an A-line skirt and boots. To dress it up for evening, remove the turtleneck, add a dressier belt, pants and sandals. Pretty earrings and swept-back hair add some polish.

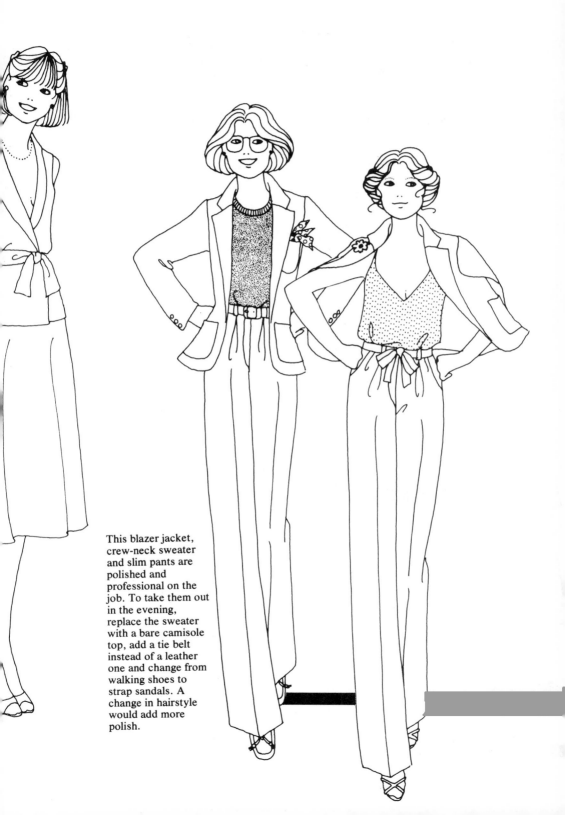

This blazer jacket, crew-neck sweater and slim pants are polished and professional on the job. To take them out in the evening, replace the sweater with a bare camisole top, add a tie belt instead of a leather one and change from walking shoes to strap sandals. A change in hairstyle would add more polish.

## Shopping Tips for Working Women

One reason working women often have "what to wear" problems is the lack of time to shop. With busy jobs, often combined with a family, you just can't browse through store after store looking for what you want. Here are some ideas that can make shopping easier.

■ Get in the habit of shopping for several things at once. The best time is before each change of season. Assess what you'll need as specifically as you can, make a list, right down to the color and fabric you'd like. Then shop.

■ Shop at the beginning of the season. Stores have the best selection then and you'll be most likely to find the size, color, and style you want.

■ Try to find a couple of manufacturers that have your kind of clothes, then look for all the stores that stock them. You can even write the manufacturer and ask for a list of stores near you that carry these clothes.

■ If you shop in a large department store, be on the lookout for special "career" shops where many kinds of clothes working women need are displayed. More and more department stores are realizing there is a need for one centralized shopping location that minimizes walking around the store.

■ Ask if the department stores in your city have personalized shopping services of any kind and take advantage of them. Some stores offer one salesperson who will follow you from department to department so you don't have to look for sales help in each place you shop.

■ If you find a store and a department that works for you, befriend one of the salespersons and ask her to let you know when things come in that fit your needs.

■ Be aware that many small boutiques cater to a particular kind of shopper. If you find the boutique that caters to your kind of need, your shopping is simplified.

■ Do have a charge where you shop. It makes buying and returning, when necessary, much faster. You can usually just call and have something you may have seen advertised charged and sent, then picked up if it is necessary to return it, all without you having set foot in the store.

## WHAT TO WEAR WHEN YOU'RE IN THE SPOTLIGHT

One of the happiest occurrences today is the increased visibility of women speaking in public, both on television and in front of live audiences of all kinds, from groups of their professional peers to political or community affairs groups. This presents a whole new set of ''what to wear'' questions.

### The "Public" Look to Aim For

If you're going to be doing the talking, you want people to concentrate on what you're saying, not on how you look. Aim for a classic, feminine, and flattering look. A shirtwaist dress, a suit, a silk shirt and skirt, and for less formal talks, a shirt and tailored pants would all work well. Stay away from fussy details that are distracting: no busy prints or large patterns, no bows at the neck or low, low necklines, no jewelry that dangles or tempts you to play with it, no bracelets that clank as you gesture. You'll find that anything with pockets is a plus. You can slip your hand in gracefully instead of fidgeting; you can also keep index cards with notes on them tucked in a pocket, ready to be pulled out should you need them.

99

Television has some special dos and don'ts. Don't wear anything with sharp color contrasts such as black and white or beige and dark brown. Color contrasts tend to "jump" on camera. Big patterns also tend to jump and become distracting. Anything that glitters, such as a big gold pin or sparkly stones, will be distracting, too.

Television stations are usually very cooperative and will provide you with as much information ahead of time as possible. It's to their advantage as well as yours that all goes well. Here's a checklist to run down with station personnel a day or so before you appear.

## TV CHECKLIST

■ Will you be standing or sitting? (If you're sitting, be sure your skirt "sits" well and doesn't pull or fall open. Pants are a good choice for sitting.)

■ If there are other guests, what will they be wearing?

■ Is the lighting direct or overhead and what tips do they offer for making-up?

■ What color is the background? (You don't want to clash with it.)

■ Ask if you can come to the studio ahead of time to check out your hair, makeup and clothes under simulated conditions. It's often possible for you to see yourself on a monitor.

## Hair and Makeup

Both your hair and makeup should be as simple and flattering as possible. Don't pick a fussy or exaggerated hairstyle or overdo makeup. Do remember, however, that your face will probably be reduced to a couple of inches on the TV screen and in a public hall you'll be far from your audience. Makeup that's a bit more definite than that for ordinary streetwear is in order. You should apply just a bit more blusher and lip color or pick a slightly brighter shade. If your brows are pale, darken them just a bit with a soft pencil or a powder brow preparation.

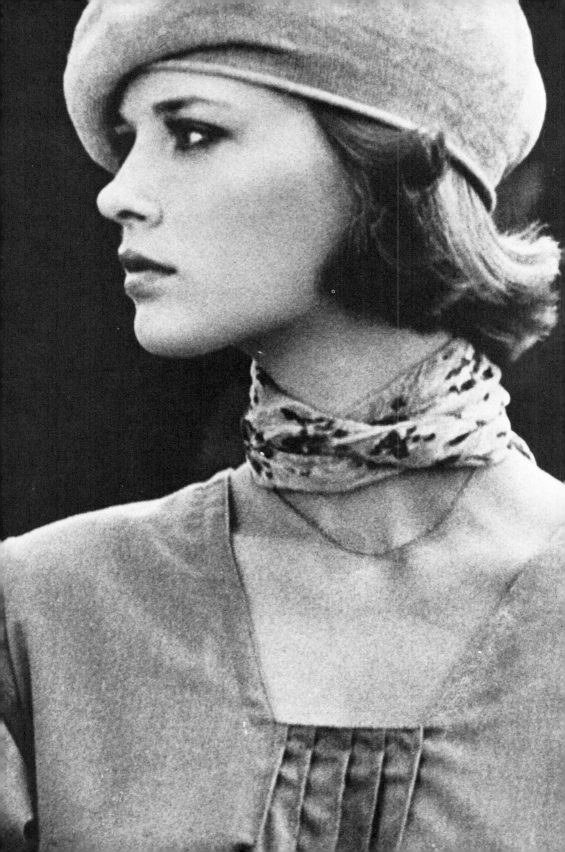

THE POLISH

# 5
# How to be a good shopper

M ost of us fall into one of two broad categories when it comes to shopping: you enjoy it and find it a pleasant, almost sensual experience, or you dislike it, putting it off whenever possible. The reasons you like or dislike shopping are probably more subtle than you imagine. If you dislike it, you may tell yourself it's because you don't have the time, the stores are crowded or you can never find what you want. This may all be true, but since these are easily solvable problems, which you haven't managed to solve, they probably have less to do with why you dislike shopping than some of the subtle psychological attitudes you bring to it. Even if you like to shop, you may still be a poor shopper, spending your money unwisely on things that don't satisfy your real needs. If you see yourself constantly in any of the shopping patterns below, you need to change your habits and, in some cases, the way you see yourself. You'll find a lot of help in this chapter.

## The Impulsive Shopper*

You like to shop, but you need instant gratification. You will probably end up buying something, whether you need it or not. If you can't find what you came for—or if you had no particular purchase in mind—you will undoubtedly come across something so enticing or that is such a

* From "How to Be a Better Shopper Than You Ever Were Before" by Lila Nadell, *Glamour*, April 1979.

106

good buy, you just have to have it. Need or use often
have little to do with your purchases. You often shop to
relieve frustration or a feeling of powerlessness. You are
also the dream of all retailers. They set up entire departments to appeal to your psychological needs. You are also
likely to be the woman who complains of nothing to wear.
You have a closet full of items none of which seem to
have a working relationship to each other.

You can become a better shopper by disciplining yourself to stay out of stores unless you have a particular
purchase in mind. Before you actually go out to shop, try
to be as specific about the item as possible. For example,
if you need a blouse, decide what things you want to wear
it with, what color and basic style would be best, and
about how much you want to pay. Then go directly
to the blouse department and look for blouses that fit
your needs. You will also find it helpful to do some soul-
searching to find out what is frustrating you and sending
you to stores to find the satisfactions that are missing
somewhere else in your life. A new, more rewarding job
or a change in a personal relationship may be what you
really need.

## The Indecisive Shopper

You probably don't like shopping because you find it difficult to make up your mind without someone else's help.
A friend or the salesperson frequently makes decisions
for you. Indecision often follows you out of the store and
lingers long enough to send you back next day to return
your purchase, buy something else and perhaps repeat the
whole maneuver again. This shopper generally suffers
from low self-esteem and a poor self-image. Anyone else's
opinion is valued more than your own and you may also
have internalized someone else's view of you—often a
husband's or mother's.

You may find it helpful to do some thinking about what

kind of things you really like and feel comfortable in, then go out and buy them. The more you learn to develop your own sense of style and taste, the less you'll feel compelled to rely on someone else's.

## The Status Shopper

Nothing but the best will do for you, which is fine, if you can afford it and if what is reputed to be "the best" really is. If you can buy designer labels or status-store clothes, you are getting good merchandise, but you may be paying a lot more than necessary. Psychologically, what's going on here is a lack of self-worth. You don't trust yourself to make wise choices about what to buy so you put your trust in a store name or a label.

You can solve a lot of problems by learning what real quality in clothes is. (We'll discuss this later in the chapter.) Once you feel secure in knowing what you're buying, it will have the subtle psychological effect of boosting your ego while making you able to rely on your own choices rather than on the real or imagined status of someone else's.

## The Class-Conscious Shopper

You are the opposite of the Status Shopper. You tend to shop in discount stores and low-end chain stores regardless of what you can afford. You do this because you feel uncomfortable and out of place in more exclusive or elegant stores. You are likely to be easily intimidated by salespersons in better stores, feeling they know you don't belong as soon as you step inside. What you're expressing with this kind of shopping pattern is a low estimate of yourself. Your self-image is poor. You may also feel that if you look well-dressed and prosperous, people will expect more of you and you won't be able to deliver.

To change your shopping pattern, you need to change

your mind set. You need to begin consciously thinking of yourself as someone who deserves more and who is able to handle it. Forcing yourself to upgrade your choice of store may make you nervous at first, but the better merchandise and the more pleasant shopping atmosphere can win out, if you let it. Probably the most useful thing you can do is to examine your budget and see if it's really necessary to shop so "poorly." If it's not, this clearly points out that something besides necessity is driving you. This can be a big step toward changing the pattern.

## The Faddist Shopper

You probably love shopping because it gives you an opportunity to establish an identity. What you are usually looking for is something that is so offbeat it calls attention to yourself. Psychologically, you feel you will only be noticed and "count" because of what you have on. What you have to offer as a person just isn't enough. You are the one who does most to help new styles catch on because the fashion industry can always count on you to appear in whatever is newest. You run the risk of choosing styles that are here one minute and gone the next and of picking something so far out people question your judgment.

To become a better shopper, try to resist the urge to be the first to own everything. Let someone else be the guinea pig for a change and you sit back and evaluate what you *really* think of the look. This will help you develop some judgmental skills and it will save you a lot of money on the fads your good sense tells you to pass up. Over a period of time, it will also demonstrate that you have a lot more going for you than what's on your back. Not making yourself so visible for negative reasons will give others a chance to appreciate you for more positive attributes.

## The Cautious Shopper

You're dead opposite to the Faddist. You won't buy anything unless the whole crowd owns it. The old adage, "there's safety in numbers" was made for you. One of two things is going on here psychologically. You are either so afraid of standing out you go out of your way to conform or you want so badly to "belong" that you go out of your way to look like everyone else. Either way, you are telling the world that you are afraid of risks, unassertive, and possibly dull. From a clothes point of view, you're not getting your money's worth. By the time you feel comfortable buying a new look, everyone else is on to something new, always leaving you one step behind.

You probably accept the role of follower because you are afraid of rejection. If you concentrate on developing your own sense of style, you will find your fear of rejection fading. Once you know yourself and what you like, what everyone else is wearing won't seem so compelling. You will be dressing to please yourself and to gain your own goals rather than dressing to look like everyone else.

## The Bargain Shopper

You aren't to be confused with the Class-Conscious Shopper who looks only for inexpensive merchandise or with the Status Shopper who wants the best for the most. The Bargain Shopper wants the best, but at a special price because it's necessary for you to think of yourself as a special person. Being able to find the best at a better price could be your way of telling the world how bright you are. Your reward for the many hours you spend shopping is a reaffirmation of your self-esteem and the respect you feel friends give you for having made this great buy.

The pitfall here is the inordinate amount of time you have to spend uncovering your buys. You also risk buying something that's not useful to you just because you think it's such a good buy. Psychologically, you need to realize that there are many other more constructive ways of being special. Being good at your job, achieving personal goals, just having people respond positively to you can all be ways in which you are special, and they are more meaningful than just being the best bargain hunter on the block.

## IMPROVING YOUR SKILLS

Betty, a young woman who lives in a large city with all kinds of shopping opportunities had a problem many women share. Fall was approaching and she had a new, more demanding job that called for the right clothes to set the tone and project her new image. Betty began poking through her closet to take stock of things. By chance, she happened on an idea that could work well for you. As she was pulling things out, mostly with an eye to which ones needed to go to the cleaner, she realized that she didn't like much of what she was sorting through enough to be bothered with cleaning. Considering what her budget would allow for new buys, she felt discouraged; she needed too much, and she couldn't afford to make mistakes with a new job image at stake. She started to pull out clothes and put those she called "winners" in one pile and those she called "losers" in another. The winners were things she felt comfortable in and at ease with, and in this case, looked right for the new job. The losers were things she didn't like and hadn't worn much for one reason or another. Next, she tried to see what about the winners made them work and what about the losers made them fail. She discovered that most of her winners were in the beige and brown family—which looked well with her blond complexion—and they had classic, simple lines. The losers tended to be in dramatic colors—which probably looked enticing in the store—that she didn't feel comfortable with, or faddy, trendy styles that seemed out-of-date now. If she used what she'd learned about her taste in style and color as a guide when she shopped, she

111

knew she'd do much better than she had before. You might try going through your own closet and see what you discover about yourself. How many things did you buy emotionally because of color lure or a style you couldn't resist or because you simply didn't stop to think how many occasions you'd have to wear a particular blouse or dress?

While you have everything pulled out of your closet, do some rethinking about what you like. Can you put any of these things together differently so that you get more looks from them? Could you add a new accessory or two to get more potential from what you already own?

You can improve your shopping skills by taking a lesson from professional buyers. Before they make purchases for their stores, they "shop the market." They go from manufacturer to manufacturer to see what's being offered—what styles, what colors, how things are put together, what the prices are. You can do the same. If you're about to say you don't have time to shop with no intention of buying, ask yourself a few questions: How often do you usually shop and how much time do you spend at it? How successful is your average shopping trip? Have you lived happily ever after with your buys or did too many have to be returned? It's a pretty safe bet that the answers to these questions will make you decide it's worth taking a morning or afternoon to shop around and get a feeling for what's available. This trip can also have a lot of psychological benefits. This is the time to forget all your usual shopping hang-ups—because this time, you're not really buying. Don't be afraid to go into the most expensive stores or departments. Try on whatever you see that interests you, regardless of style or price, and forget all your preconceived ideas of what you can and can't wear. You may be in for some surprises once you actually try something on without the pressure of deciding whether or not you're going to buy it. This can be a wonderful learning experience that will help you establish a strong personal style.

In addition to shopping the market, you might also shop the magazines. Look through the fashion magazines you trust and see what's being worn and how things are put together and add this to the information you got from your

---

## SEVEN IN-STORE TIPS
## FOR THE SMART SHOPPER

Once you're actually in a store ready to buy, here are some things you should think about before you plunk down your money.

1 Be sure the item you're buying satisfies a need, not just a want. (Unless you've already satisfied all your needs and have some cash left over.)

2 Be sure the color works with most things you want to wear with it.

3 If you're buying something to go with a specific skirt, blouse or pants, be sure you have that item with you. Unless you see both pieces together, they can miss in color or proportion.

4 Don't buy unless you're satisfied with these four things: price, fit, style, and color.

5 When you try something on, move around a bit, make sure it sits well, that it looks well from all angles, and most of all, that you feel comfortable in it.

6 Don't buy it if you feel, "Oh, well, I can always take it back." You may not have the energy and this purchase will probably end up in your "losers" pile next year.

7 If something costs more than you feel you want to pay, but satisfies a need well, see if you can make this purchase do double duty, maybe for day and evening, so you can eliminate something else, or if you can, buy something else you need for a little less than you planned to spend.

---

preshopping expedition. Now go through your wardrobe and decide what you really need to buy, what color you think you want, and a good idea of how you'd like it to look. Think back to where you saw things that attracted you, and return to these stores armed with some very precise ideas about what you want and what you know exists. We'll bet you do your total shopping in less time and with more success than you've had before!

## HOW TO RECOGNIZE QUALITY IN CLOTHES

No matter what you can afford to pay for something, you want to get the most for your money. To do this, you have to be able to spot quality—or the lack of it. Once you become a pro at this, you can take advantage of a good buy, even in discount and outlet shops, because you know what you're getting. Knowing quality when you see it frees you from always having to pay more at classy stores or for name labels. It allows you to rely on your own ability to select quality merchandise instead of someone else's.

Though you can't buy a gorgeous pure silk satin dress for nothing, quality does come at all prices. You can get top quality at top prices, but you can also often get something comparable for a lot less. Consider this experience, shared by two sisters. Jane and Victoria both lived in the suburbs and liked to meet for lunch and some shopping in the city. Victoria usually shopped at elegant boutiques or the big, classy department stores in town. Although Jane liked to browse in these stores, she often did her buying in mass volume stores or in discount chains. Jane and her husband were saving for a Caribbean vacation in February and she didn't want to spend too much on fall clothes, so when Victoria suggested they do the boutiques, Jane said, no. "Well, I'm not going to settle for the junk that's in those stores you like to shop in," Victoria answered. Her statement sounded defensive to Jane, so she suggested that Victoria learn how to spot a good buy no

114

matter where it's offered. An hour later, they were trying on skirts and Victoria was about to buy one for $75 when Jane showed her something similar for $50. Jane pointed out to Victoria that both skirts were good quality wool, a plus. The more expensive one was fully lined while the cheaper one was lined only in back. Jane pointed out that in this case, the cheaper one was a better idea. The lining was in the back where it was needed to help the skirt keep its shape, and since the skirt was a wrap style, the friction of the two unlined pieces in front kept them from opening up and exposing too much leg. The lining of the fully lined skirt slipped on itself and the front opened up exposing leg, slip, and whatever else was being worn. The more expensive skirt had two pockets, one in each side seam, useful if you're in the habit of putting your hands in your pockets or carrying a tissue, but adding nothing to the look of the skirt. The cheaper one had no pockets. Since Victoria really didn't care about the pockets, the extra expense they represented wasn't something she needed to pay for. Victoria bought the cheaper skirt and found a great buy on a shirt to wear with it for $25!

We're not suggesting you turn yourself into a Bargain Shopper, as described a few pages back. We are suggesting that you may very often be paying for things you neither want or need, such as the lining and the pockets in this skirt, or worse yet, paying for something you aren't really getting—good quality.

## DON'T BELIEVE EVERYTHING YOU'VE ALWAYS HEARD

You've probably heard that anything made of "all wool," "all silk" or "all cotton" was quality. There are many grades of these fabrics, from poor to excellent, and the fact that they are not combined with a synthetic fiber isn't always good. Synthetics can often add to the wearability and comfort of a garment. Cheaper grades of any fabric tend to "pill," that is tiny balls of yarn appear on the surface of the fabric during wear. To test for this, rub your finger vigorously over an inconspicuous spot and see if any pills appear. Remember that, in general, the lighter the weight of a fabric, the more fragile it is and the more likely it will show signs of wear or need special care.

Supply and demand greatly affect the price of a fabric but have nothing to do with its quality. For years rayon was not in demand and was therefore inexpensive. Now rayon is experiencing a comeback and is in greater demand—and consequently is wearing a higher price tag. None of this affects the quality of what your dollar is buying. The lesson here is that if you're buying an "in" fabric, you're probably paying a little extra for the fact that it's trendy.

You may also have heard that the more fabric a garment contains, the better its quality. This is really not true now —if it ever was. Although more expensive garments usually have more generous seam allowances and deeper hems, this represents such a small difference in total fabric, it doesn't affect the cost of the garment greatly. Style is the big determinant here. If styles are for big voluminous skirts and tops, that's what you'll find most of, and because they do require more yardage, they may be more expensive than in previous years when clothes weren't so full. If, as has happened recently, clothes slim down after a period of being full, you won't see much decrease in price as a result of the decrease in yardage. Inflation usually pushes prices up bit by bit each year, regardless of style changes.

If all this leaves you feeling that fabric is, at best, a chancy guide to quality, you're right. Although good quality should always mean good fabric, there are other quality indicators easier for a novice to spot. If these are present, you can usually assume the fabric is good quality, too. A manufacturer will not usually go to the trouble and expense of putting quality craftsmanship into a garment made of poor fabric.

116

Buying designer labels as quality assurance is another hazy area for the average consumer. We have already pointed out that you very often pay more for the chic of a particular designer label and although you do usually get quality, you can often duplicate that quality and much of the same look at a lower price. Many women are aware of this and shy away from *all* designer labels. This can be a mistake. Remember that there are some designers that pride themselves on producing good quality clothes at reasonable prices. Do buy these labels. The ones to be suspicious of are those so highly publicized that their name appears on everything from towels to underwear. Somehow or other, the consumer is going to pay for all that publicity, and though the name does represent a dependable design talent, you may not care to pay for all the extra hoopla that surrounds the name.

## SUREFIRE QUALITY GUIDES

These are the dependable indicators of quality that any woman can easily learn to spot:

■ Check to see that thread, zipper, and lining color are good matches to the garment's fabric.

■ Look for clean, threadfree buttonholes that fit button size well. Look for seams that are finished well—raw edges pinked—or better yet, overcast with small stitches close together to prevent raveling.

■ Check outside leg seam in pants. If it's pressed flat, you're looking at quality construction that insures pants will hang well.

■ Check detailing like topstitching, flaps on pockets, and pocket edges. Is detailing well done, stitching neat and free of threads, pocket edges securely attached?

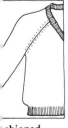
shioned
r sleeve

■ When buying a sweater, look for full-fashioned sleeves. You can identify them by tiny stitch marks

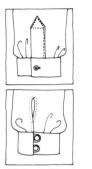

High-quality sleeve
cuff construction

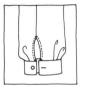

Poor-quality sleeve
cuff construction

outlining the sleeve where it is attached to garment. Cuffs and waistband should be knitted on rather than stitched on. This gives the sweater a better shape, especially after washing or dry cleaning.

■ Check the opening of long-sleeved blouses. A nice neat placket indicates quality. An opening formed by leaving the last few inches of the under-arm seam open indicates poor quality.

■ Check the lining when buying a coat. In quality coats, the coat hem is caught to the lining hem rather than being sewn to the coat fabric. This gives a soft rolled finish rather than a flat one. Another acceptable construction is a closed bottom where lining is hemmed to coat hem. If the lining hangs completely free, the coat construction leaves something to be desired.

■ If a skirt or dress is hemmed with clear plastic thread, watch out. This kind of stitching pulls out quickly and indicates the manufacturer probably used other poor construction techniques.

■ In garments with plaids, stripes, or large patterns, be sure the seams are matched well.

## HOW TO READ AN AD

Advertising is part of our daily lives. A good ad can lead you quickly to what you're looking for, saving you hours of scouting around trying to locate it. An ad can also have the same psychological effect on you as can merchandise in a store. Beware the impulse to rush off and buy something just because the ad looked appealing—especially if you tend to be an Impulsive Shopper. Ads announcing sales are probably the trickiest to deal with because they often use terms that many people don't understand clearly. These terms are used consistently in ads for all kinds of merchandise, so learning them can help shopping all across the board. Here are some you should become familiar with.

Sale: This means that the regular merchandise of the store is marked down. Often a specific percentage such as ten or twenty percent will be deducted from all sale items.

Special purchase: This is new merchandise brought into the store for the purpose of a sale. Although you can often get good values, be cautious. Special purchase merchandise is sometimes of poorer quality than that which the store usually carries or it may be something a manufacturer couldn't sell so the store got a good buy. Just be sure you look carefully at what you're buying.

Clearance sale: This is usually a reduction in price on merchandise previously offered at a higher price by the store. Don't expect new merchandise; in fact, clearance merchandise usually consists of items that have been around a while and though you can often get spectacular buys, count on a pressing or cleaning job.

Comparable value: The advertised item is similar to but not identical to merchandise selling at a "comparable" price. The ad usually reads something like this: silk shirts, $25, comparable value $40. You can often get a good buy, but do check out quality points to make sure you're aware of what you're getting.

Liquidation sale: This implies the retailer is going out of business and wants to liquidate all the merchandise he has. There's nothing wrong with this kind of sale as long as it *is* a true liquidation sale. Many small shops have been having liquidation sales for years; it's their standard way of doing business and it's generally suspect. Shops that continually have liquidation sales often offer second-class merchandise at more than first-class prices.

Clearance center: Many large department stores have a permanent location in the store—sometimes it's a separate building or warehouse—where you can find clearance merchandise. The items sold here have been in regular stock and aside from being manhandled, they can be good buys. In such a center, you'll usually find everything from appliances to clothes.

Irregular: Merchandise offered as irregular is probably the trickiest for an unaware consumer to take advantage of. You know the merchandise isn't perfect, and it can often be a challenge to find out what's wrong with it. If you notice large imperfections—holes, runs, snags—you can easily decide that this isn't what you're looking for. If, as is usually the case, you can't immediately spot the problem, you know it's there and you need to locate it so you can determine if it will affect the wear or ultimately the look of the garment. Salespeople will sometimes help if they know that most of the merchandise has a particular kind of imperfection. Examples of slight irregularities can be a print that's slightly off in one spot, a knit with a few pulled stitches, a color that's not quite even over the entire garment. Most of these things aren't serious or even noticeable unless you're looking for them, but don't settle on a buy unless you've found the irregularity and can live with it. If you're shopping in a discount or chain store, you can often get a very good buy on a slightly irregular designer item. The high standards and prices of the designer may force him to reject even the slightest imperfection, so these garments are sold to discount stores. The label is usually cut out so that the designer's name isn't obvious. A garment with a label deliberately cut to obliterate the designer's name is often an indication you're getting a good buy.

Second: This is a broad term that indicates merchandise is not perfect. It usually is used for merchandise with more obvious defects than "irregular" but this is not always true. Look carefully before buying seconds.

## YOUR RIGHTS AS A SHOPPER

You will have better luck solving your shopping problems if you have some idea of what you can and can't expect when something you bought doesn't work out as you had hoped. The most tempting approach when a purchase goes wrong is to get justifiably angry and shout and pound your fist. This approach usually doesn't work well; it turns off the person you're yelling at, making him or her less sympathetic to your problem. It's best to be firm but polite. It's also best to start by taking your complaint to someone in authority so you don't have to repeat your story several times, getting angrier with each repetition. Ask for the department supervisor or the store manager, if it's a small shop, and start there. If it's a large department store and you get nowhere in the department where you purchased the item, ask if they have an adjustment department—most do—and take your complaint there.

## VALID COMPLAINTS

In general, if you bought something of reasonable quality and if after the first washing or dry cleaning, provided you followed instructions for care, your garment performs disappointingly, you have a valid complaint. Take it back and be prepared to point out the problem quickly. Fading, shrinking, raveling, losing shape are all examples of legitimate complaints. Don't be afraid to complain about merchandise bought on sale. Just because something is reduced doesn't mean you can't expect it to wear decently. If you bought something tagged "as is" or "damaged," that's a different story.

If you purchased something in one store and find it considerably cheaper at another, it's worth going to the first store with some proof that the exact item is being sold for less somewhere else. Many stores will refund you the difference because it's bad public relations to have you thinking they jack up prices astronomically.

121

Almost any reputable store has a refund policy that allows you to return undamaged merchandise within a certain period of time. If you're shopping in a chain or discount store, you'll often find their policy on refunds posted near the door. If not, ask. Be sure you know what is required in the way of a sales slip and intact tickets on the garment. Many women find having a charge account simplifies returns and refunds. If you have a charge, you can almost always get a garment credited to your account, even in stores that have a policy of no cash refunds. If you have no charge, you get a credit to apply to new purchases, but you can't get your money back. Many stores also have time limits on refunds, especially discount stores, so be sure you know how long you may keep something and still return it.

## MAIL-ORDER SHOPPING

Over 30 billion dollars worth of goods was sold through the mail last year. Of course not all of it was clothing, but clothing does account for a sizable chunk of this figure. In addition to the catalogs of large mail-order chains, there are hundreds of small national and local mail-order houses that sell first quality merchandise. It's an appealing way to shop because you don't have to step outside your door. Decisions are simplified because the choices are limited. Orders are filled promptly, usually within thirty days, often much less, as now stipulated by laws regulating mail-order selling (or whatever time is stated in the mail-order offer), and if you don't receive your order within this time, the seller is obligated to notify you, telling you exactly when you can expect delivery.

If you keep a few things in mind about style and fit, you can use mail-order shopping to simplify your life. When buying clothes, look for the following kind of details which minimize fit problems and the possibility of return.

■ Look for elasticized or drawstring waists.

■ Pick a wrap style when possible.

■ Avoid things with definite waistlines.

■ Items sized S M L usually have no complicated fit problems. S is usually an 8-10; M is 12-14; L is 16. This is a general rule, many mail-order houses break down sizing details in the front or back of their catalogs, so check this out before you order.

■ Pick dependable colors such as navy, brown, wine, gray, black, and white. Then there'll be no surprises about what "teal" or "chartreuse" or other less specific colors may turn out to be.

# 6

# How to organize your closet

## and your clothes thinking

A well-organized, well-thought-out closet can make the problems of what to wear when much easier. Unless you've already perfected the art of organization, you've undoubtedly spent some frustrating minutes standing in front of your closet trying to find the peach blouse that goes with the rust skirt. After a few futile attempts, you're likely to chuck it and settle for the old faithful beige dress you wore yesterday because it's right there in the front of the closet where you hung it last night. If you're wise enough to realize the importance of clothes in creating the kind of self-image you want, it's foolish to make less than optimum use of the clothes you own just because your closet is a disaster.

Organizing your closet is a simple and self-perpetuating process. Once you've really lived with an organized closet, you won't be able to stand a messy one again. We suggest this organizational idea for several reasons. First hang similar things together: all the blouses, all the skirts, and do the same with pants and jackets. Keep color and mood in mind, too. For example, move from white and beiges into colors, keeping things in color families. Keep the casual things together and keep dressier ones together. One unbreakable rule—don't hang one thing over another, such as a jacket over a pair of pants or a skirt. All this may sound like an overly fastidious or even neurotic approach, but have faith. It's not. What it will do is make finding any particular thing much easier—you know a shirt *has* to be hanging with other shirts or a skirt with other skirts. Even more importantly, it will open up a

126

whole new range of put-together possibilities for you which could mean you'll end up with a lot more looks than you thought you had.

A young woman recently came into *Glamour's* offices for a fashion makeover. She had written us saying that she never seemed to have the right things to wear for her job as a teacher. She told us a few things about the clothes she owned and how much she budgeted for clothes yearly. We were interested in her and invited her to come to *Glamour* because her problems seemed to have many elements that numerous readers could relate to. We asked her to take some pictures of her clothes so we could be thinking of what we could suggest she add that would make sense for her kind of life. She photographed her clothes, laid out neatly on her bed. She also took pictures of her closet. What we observed was that she bought many separates that matched—for example, a rust-printed calico skirt and blouse and a floral-print shirt and skirt. We noticed that she photographed these items together and hung them together in her closet. We suspected that she, like many women we've run across, wore these pieces *only* with each other—the calico-print top with its matching skirt and the floral-print top with its skirt. We could see immediately from the pictures that she sent us that there were several things each of these tops and bottoms could be mixed with to give her more options. Hanging them together had been limiting her thinking about how to use them in her wardrobe. If you separate all tops and bottoms physically in your closet, it will help you to separate them emotionally and open up a new range of possibilities for all the pieces you own.

When you're organizing your closet in this way, it means you're going to have to pull everything out. As you're doing this, try to look at each item with a fresh eye. Try putting different tops with different bottoms in ways you've never combined them before. We'll bet you come up with quite a few new and successful looks. Until you get used to wearing things with different partners,

127

you might want to jot down on paper all the new, interesting combinations you come up with now so you'll remember them later.

## SPACE SAVERS AND SPACE-SAVING IDEAS THAT WORK

Every big department store has a notions department that is filled with all kinds of hangers, storage boxes and bags geared to organizing and saving space in your closet. Some of them are a waste of money—we'll get to those in a minute—but others are truly ingenious and really help you conserve space and make things easier to locate in the bargain. Here is a list of some we think are worth owning:

Multiple blouse hangers: One hanger with a half-dozen shoulder bars that hangs a half-dozen blouses, making each one easy to get at.

Multiple skirt hangers: One hanger with a half-dozen clips to hang skirts.

Multiple pants hangers: One hanger with several bars to hang pants over. Be sure you pick one where the bar unfastens, rather like the bar in a safety pin, to make it easy to slide pants on and off.

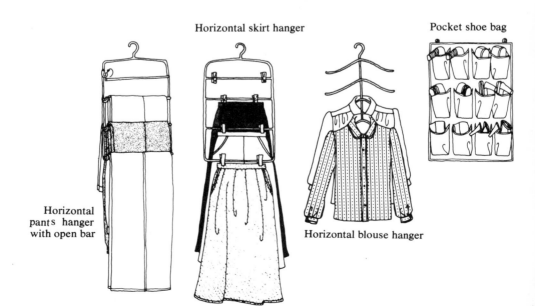

Horizontal skirt hanger

Pocket shoe bag

Horizontal pants hanger with open bar

Horizontal blouse hanger

Canvas shoe bags for door back: **Contains pockets to slip shoes in so they can be hung on the door, saving floor space, or probably more importantly, leaving floor space clean to give the psychological feeling of space.**
Clear plastic storage boxes: **Used for gloves, scarves, belts, they make things easy to spot and get to.**
Belt hooks or bar: **Either a bar with several hooks attached to it or individual hooks that can be attached to a closet door make storing and getting at belts simple.**
Battery closet light: **If your closet is small, this is a particularly good idea** because the extra light makes finding things so much easier.
Extra clothes bar: **A second bar to hang clothes on can literally double your closet space. If you have room, do install one. In some cases, you may have to move your original bar up or down to accommodate a second one, but it's worth the trouble. Put clothes used less frequently, such as off-season ones, on the most inaccessible rack.**

## CLOSET GADGETS TO AVOID

Unworkable or unnecessary gadgets in your closet not only wastes your money, they can actually reduce your clothes options. For example:
Garment bags: **Hanging things in garment bags takes up extra space in your closet—the bag is bulky—and it makes getting to the clothes in them difficult. Also, what you can't see, you're not likely to think of and wear. When it comes right down to it, there are very few things that are so fragile they need a garment bag to protect them. Make it a practice to use bags only for out-of-season clothes and try to hang the bag somewhere else so they won't confuse the issue with clothes you're wearing every day.**
Ordinary shoe boxes: **Many woman are in the habit of storing shoes or anything else that fits into them in ordinary closed shoe boxes. Because you can't see through**

the boxes, you're never sure where anything is. Since locating exactly what you're looking for is hard, you often settle for what happens to be in the box you reach for first.

<u>Floor shoe racks</u>: These racks are clumsy. You have to bend down and get your head lost in the hems hanging above to find what you want. Using a door shoe bag is simpler and leaves the floor space clear.

<u>Bar-hanging belt racks</u>: If you have the choice between a belt rack that hangs on the back of a closet door or one that hangs in the closet on the bar, pick the one that attaches to the door. The belts hanging inside the closet among the clothes are hard to get at, and you must balance the weight so the hanger doesn't tilt. Since the door type attaches firmly to the door, it doesn't present this complication.

<u>Clamp skirt hangers</u>: Hangers that clamp across the waistband of a skirt don't usually have a strong enough grip to hold one skirt firmly, and when two or more are clamped together they all get crushed. A hanger with multiple clips that allows skirts to hang one above the other is a much better idea.

One last thought. It takes a certain amount of discipline to get in the habit of using all these organizational tools and techniques. If you take the trouble to organize your closet as we've suggested and then hang things wherever your hand hits when you take something off, you're defeating your purpose. Make a real effort to keep your closet organized for a couple of months, and the benefits, we feel, will be important enough to make you want to continue.

## WEEDING OUT

One reason most people's closets are cluttered is that they contain countless garments no longer being worn. Psychologists tell us most people fall roughly into two categories—savers and weeders. We suspect that the balance is strongly in favor of the savers. There is one very simple rule of thumb that can help you become a weeder instead of a saver: If you haven't worn something for a year, you probably aren't going to wear it and it should be weeded out. This means you will need to go through your closet thoroughly at least once a year. Actually, we recommend you do it twice a year, once in the fall and again in the spring.

To show you how helpful it can be to give your closet a thorough going-over, let's run through some of the benefits. Start by pulling everything out and piling it all on your bed. As you remove things, pile them according to season, putting all the things for the coming season in one pile, all those for the past one in another. Try on *everything* that you have for the coming season. Even if you feel you definitely want to keep it, try it on anyway. As you try it on, take a good look at the dress, skirt or whatever. Does it still fit properly? If it doesn't, put it aside to have something done about the fit problem. If it cannot be fixed—it's too short for current styles and there's no hem to let down, for example—put it in the pile to toss out. If it needs new buttons, seams repaired, or the hem fixed, put it in the pile for repairs.

One of the best reasons to try on something is to see if it's "friendly." Do you feel comfortable, attractive, and happy wearing it? If you don't, and especially if you remember that you never really felt comfortable in this particular item, admit you don't like it, that it was a mistake, and heave it. Before you do, however, study it to see where you went wrong so that you won't make the same mistake again. It's very difficult for most of us to admit we made a mistake with something, but remember, taking up space with that particular item can take space away from something that is infinitely more flattering and workable. If you analyze why you made the mistake in the first place, it will reduce the chances of your doing it again.

In going through your closet, you are bound to find a

131

few things you definitely don't want to throw out, but that you really don't wear very often. These are likely to be special clothes—very dressy things, pieces oriented around a certain kind of weather or sport. You know they function, it's just that you don't need them often. It's best to find some other spot for these clothes so they don't use closet space needed for more frequently used clothes. Maybe you can fold them and put them on a high shelf or store them in luggage. Try to find some place besides your closet to keep them.

## TEMPORARY WEEDING OUT

If you're short on closet space, especially if you live in a city apartment where closet space always seems to be at a premium, it can often be worth the extra expense to take advantage of storage outside your apartment. Clothes for another season, special item clothes, or anything you won't be wearing for months, can be stored with your dry cleaner. Most neighborhood cleaners have storage facilities, often combined with dry cleaning service so that when the clothes are returned to you, they're clean and ready to wear. This service is expensive, but it can often be worth the money. If your alternative is to squeeze everything in the same closet, making it extremely difficult to find what you want because there are so many things in the way, it is worth the investment and better for all your clothes, to spend the extra money on storage. When clothes are cramped into too small a space, you usually have to press fragile things such as soft shirts or lightweight dresses every time you want to wear them. You may consider it worth a little extra money to avoid this. If you have expensive investments such as a good winter coat or a fur coat, don't cram them in your closet from season to season, at least store these few things to protect them when they are not actively in use.

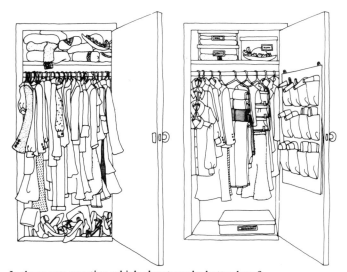

Is there any question which closet works better here?

# 7

# The
# polish
# on your
# look

Picking the right clothes for the image you want to project is obviously important, but to make the clothes really work for you, you need the right polish—hair and makeup to help you come across as attractive as well as well-dressed. Often, it's just this polish that makes the difference. You'll have no trouble understanding this if you think about the times your hair or makeup didn't please you and remember your reaction to it. "If my hair looks a mess, I feel a mess all over," is something we've all said. What's worse, we usually act out our feelings. If you think you look blah, you often act that way and other people draw conclusions about your abilities from the way you look and the subtle message you project. A recent University of Georgia study showed that both men and women judged attractive people as more skilled and more socially likeable. The study points out that this may, in fact, not be true, but if people *believe* it to be true and act on this belief, it's too important to overlook. We are exposed to this kind of thinking very early. Another study done by a group of behavior scientists showed that teachers, when assigning arbitrary grades to students they didn't know, gave the best grades to the most attractive students. Fortunately, the right clothes, hairdo, and makeup can help us all project a more attractive appearance.

## HAIR

The kind and quality of hair you have will always and forever be intimately involved with how you wear your hair. If you have thin, fine hair, you will never be able to achieve the same styles as a woman with thick, curly hair. That's just a fact of your life. Jane, who has fine, soft, brown hair was continuously trying to achieve the thick, curly, face-framing look of her sister and never succeeded. Her sister had entirely different hair—thick, coarse and naturally curly. But Jane had her "moment of truth." She says, "One day I was having my hair shampooed before getting it cut and the woman shampooing it ran her fingers through it and said, 'You have such marvelous soft hair.' I was going to object and tell her how I hated my soft hair until I noticed how thick and bushy hers was. To her, my soft, fine hair was the most marvelous thing in the world. From that day on, I decided to accept what I had and try to make it look as attractive as possible for *my* kind of hair. When I sat down to have it cut, for the first time in my life I told the hairdresser I wanted something *realistic,* something I could maintain with my kind of hair. I've had a lot fewer problems since then, I can tell you."

Jane's story points up something too many women aren't willing to accept—the limitations of their own hair. If you don't accept them, you'll force yourself to live unhappily ever after. Here are the three basic hair types and some commonsense rules for each.

### Fine Hair

This hair is almost always thin as well as fine, the two hereditary traits seem to go together. It is soft, has a lot of shine and does not hold a set well. If it is naturally curly, it tends to look fuzzy rather than definitely curly, especially in humid weather. Here are some tips for coping:

137

■ Don't wear your hair longer than chin length unless you plan to wear it up most of the time. The weight of the hair will pull out the curl.

■ Spend top dollar for a good haircut. It can make or break your look.

■ Never layer-cut your hair. If you want a soft or wispy look around your face, have the hair next to your face tapered. Tapering should start at the bangs area and continue to the ears where the hair should begin to blend in with the back.

■ Permanents, unless carefully done, can make your kind of hair frizzy, so don't experiment on yourself unless you know what you're doing. Have only the best hairdresser give you a perm if you're having one at a salon.

■ Straightening your hair to remove natural curl is not a good idea. Most fine hair won't stand up well to the strong chemicals used in this procedure.

■ Blunt-cutting the ends of your hair—that is, having your hairdresser make the final cut straight across the ends—will give your hair more bulk.

■ Use water-based conditioners. They're easily identified by their thin watery consistency as compared to thick or creamy lotions. Cream or lotion products are too heavy for your hair.

■ Use protein and body-building shampoos to help your hair hold a set better. Do be aware, though, that many of these shampoos leave a slight residue on your hair. This may necessitate more frequent shampooing.

■ Setting lotions will also help your hair hold a style better. Don't overdo them, however, or you'll end up with gummy, no-shine hair.

■ Be aware that because your hair is thin and fine, oily residue and dirt will show up faster than on thicker hair so you'll have to shampoo more often. Any kind of complicated hairstyle may require more shampooing and maintenance time than you're prepared to give.

## Medium Hair

Your hair is ideal. Its medium texture gives you few limitations. It styles well and holds a set well and you can probably wear it almost any way that flatters your particular face shape. Here are a few things to remember when you're making decisions:

■ A blunt, straight-across cut will give your hair a bulkier look.

■ An angled cut at the ends will make hair lie closer to the head.

■ If you want to add fullness, have your hair layer-cut.

■ The larger the roller you use to set your hair, the looser the set will be. Large rollers, however, do give hair a full look. Small rollers will give you a tighter, more definite curl.

■ The longer you leave rollers (or a curling iron) in your hair, the curlier your hair will get. This is true only of rollers used on dry hair. If you wet-set your hair, you'll have to leave rollers in until hair is dry. The size of your roller is important to the finished look in this case.

## Coarse Hair

This kind of hair is usually thick as well as coarse, although there are more exceptions here than there are in the case of thin/fine. Your hair can look bushy if it's not styled carefully.

■ Don't have hair blunt-cut. This will only make your hair look bushy.

■ Don't have your hair cut too short, it will be hard to control—unless you want a curly cap achieved with natural curl or a perm. In this case, hair should be carefully cut and kept quite short.

■ Don't use setting lotions to add body. You already have enough.

■ A cream rinse or softening conditioner will help control your hair.

■ Don't leave electric rollers or curling irons in your hair long. You'll get too much curl and an unruly look.

■ If your hair is curly and you straighten it, be certain you condition it properly afterward. If you don't you'll end up with coarse, textured straw.

## The Right Hairstyle

Within the length and layering limitations for your hair type, there are also certain basic styles that offer versatility and attractiveness. The sketches here show you some that are contemporary.

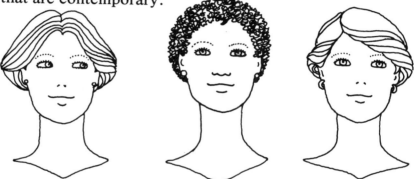

This is a good basic short cut that can be parted in the center or on the side. It's not layered, it's tapered, so it works especially well for fine hair. It will require little maintenance, so it's good for a working woman. It does require a good cut every six weeks or so.

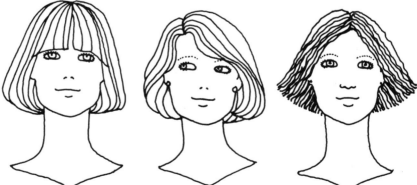

This is an attractive chin-length cut that is good for almost any hair texture. The side pieces can be either longer or shorter than the back, or hair can be the same length all around. This changes the basic look ever so slightly. Maintenance is easy; cutting is needed about every two months.

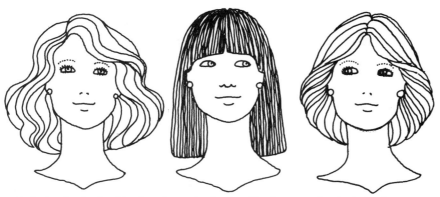

This is the classic shoulder-length cut. Again, the side pieces can be shorter or longer, depending on your taste and face shape. If they are short, as in these sketches, you can style the sides and bangs to be brushed back, giving the hair a fresh, contemporary look.

If you wear your hair longer than shoulder length you must expect to spend a fair amount of time maintaining it, depending on how often you need to shampoo it and how much drying time your particular texture requires. If you work, you will probably find that this hairstyle is just too much trouble. It also doesn't look professional, if it's too long, unless it's worn up.

## Coloring Your Hair

Highlighting the color of your hair with streaks or tinting it all over can be a good idea if you follow a few basic tips:

■ Don't change the color of your hair radically. It won't be flattering to your skin tone. Two shades darker or lighter are the best choices.

■ Try on a wig in a color close to what you're considering to get an idea whether you'll be happy with the color change.

■ If you want the look of lighter hair, but not the maintenance of tinting, consider streaking. Streaks are usually placed close to the face and are several shades lighter than your natural color. They give an all-over lighter appearance. Streaks last for three to four months. Hair

141

that's tinted all over needs redoing every three to four weeks.

■ Coloring your hair in any way means you'll have to condition it more frequently. Remember this when you're considering how much extra maintenance the color job will require. For streaked hair, plan to condition every four to five weeks. Tinted hair will probably need it every three to four weeks.

■ Henna is a popular hair coloring idea at present. It is often used to give dark hair reddish highlights. If used properly, it can be very attractive. Have a good salon do the job and remember to condition your hair monthly afterward because henna is drying. Henna highlights last for about four months and are considered "permanent" coloring.

## Dos and Don'ts for Healthy, Happy Hair

DON'T use two chemical processes such as coloring and a permanent. The combination of both will damage all but the strongest hair.

DO relax about how frequently you have to shampoo your hair. Even daily shampooing won't harm your hair as long as you use a mild shampoo. It is wise, however, to limit your use of heat appliances to about three times a week. You might use your dryer on the cool setting or let your hair dry naturally whenever you have the time.

DON'T spend long hours outdoors in the sun without protecting your hair with a scarf or hat of some kind. This is especially important in the summer or if your work keeps you outdoors a lot.

DO spend the time to learn to style your hair successfully yourself. If you can't blow-dry your hair well, get your hairdresser to give you some pointers. If your hair doesn't look almost as good when you do it as when you come from your favorite salon, you're doing something wrong. Anyone can learn to do a simple, handsome style well.

DON'T be afraid to tell your hairdresser *exactly* what you want. If you leave it all up to him or her, you're leaving yourself open to all kinds of problems. You will establish a better relationship between the two of you and end up with happier results if you learn to speak up.

## MAKEUP

"I feel insecure about what to use so I think it's simpler not to get involved," says one woman. Another says, "I don't want to look overdone and rather than risk that, I don't use much of anything except a little lipstick and blusher." Many women feel overwhelmed by all the color and product options available today. But as with most options, it's better to have them than not. You just have to learn what the options can do for you so you can make wise decisions.

### Color Options

The makeup options that frighten women most are those of color because they are so visible. But because they *are* so visible, they have the potential to be the most valuable. Let's start with the most basic color option, your foundation.

### Foundations

■ Let your skin tone guide you. Anything too far removed from your natural coloring will look artificial and made up. Never go more than two shades lighter or darker than your natural skin tone.

■ If you're not happy with your skin tone, if perhaps it's too ruddy or too sallow to suit you, foundation can help compensate, but stay within a shade or two of your natural tone. If your skin is sallow, warm it up a bit with a

143

foundation that has a bit of pink or peach in it. If you are already too ruddy, don't pick something too pale to compensate, just pick a color close to your own tone that has no trace of pink or peach in it. A color in the beige family is what you want. A saleswoman can be helpful here so don't be afraid to ask. Test the foundation on your face, not on your hand. The chin or forehead is a good testing spot.

## Blusher

■ A tawny blush is the safest choice because it works for almost all skin tones and it looks natural and flattering. The paler your skin and the lighter your hair, the softer the tawny blush you should pick. Dark-skinned, dark-haired women look well in deep tawny shades.
■ Pink or peach tones are another option for fair-skinned, fair-haired women. Be careful not to pick something *too* pink. You'll end up looking like a China doll. Pinks and peaches are good evening options. Look for soft, not harsh colors and blend them carefully.
■ Wine or burgundy colors are a nice change of pace for medium to dark-skinned women with darker hair. Pick soft shades for day and save the deeper ones for evening. Again, be sure you blend the color well.

## Eyeshadow

The situation here is a bit more complicated, but these tips are pretty foolproof:
■ Don't match your eye color. It looks too obvious. A color in the same family or something entirely different is more interesting.
■ Instead, pick up a color you're wearing close to your face. Try to find an eye shadow in the same color family, again, not a dead match. For example, if you're wearing a forest green sweater, a deep, smoky green shadow

144

would be pretty. A deep earth-colored shadow would go well with a rust or orange sweater. Experiment a bit until you begin to get a feeling for what goes with what.

■ Another option that works well for many women for daytime wear is simply to pick a brownish or earth-toned shadow and use it very subtly to define the shape of the eye. This way it gives the eye emphasis without really suggesting a color. Brown, bronze, earth, or mauve are good tones for this. Be sure you blend the shadow so that all you see is the subtlest hint of color.

■ A good rule of thumb for a simple and flattering method of application is this: Apply your shadow in the crease of the lid so that it imitates the curve of your brow. The two curves, one beneath the other, are flattering.

## Lipstick

■ Keep your lipcolor in the same family as your blush. If you're wearing a tawny blush, pick a tawny lipcolor. You can pick something lighter or deeper, just keep the whole palette in the same color family.

■ Colored lip glosses give you only the suggestion of color and many women find them good for daytime wear. You should still keep them in the same color family as your blush.

## Product Options

Walk past any cosmetic counter and you realize that finding a foundation, a blush, or a lipstick is not just a simple matter of color choice. There are creams, gels, powders, lotions, and a dozen other options to pick from. Sometimes it's purely a matter of personal preference, but at other times, the kind of product is very important. Here are some things to remember:

■ Your skin type can be a good guide to picking products. If your skin is oily, gels, powders, and water-based

145

formulations are your best choice. If your skin is dry, cream, lotion, and oil-based formulations are best. It's simple enough to tell whether an eye shadow or blusher is a cream or powder, but foundations can be tricky, especially the liquid ones, because you may not be able to tell whether what you're buying is water or oil-based. In general, the creamier the consistency of a foundation, the more oil it probably contains. By contrast, the more "watery" it is, the less oil it contains. If you're in doubt, ask the salesperson for advice. You may also find a foundation with an "oil blotting" ingredient, helpful if your skin is oily.

■ Check the consistency of a product. Eye shadow, blushers, and foundations come in a whole range of consistencies from thick and opaque to light and sheer. In general, the sheerer a product is, the easier it is to apply and the more natural it looks. Creams, lotions, and gels can all be either opaque or sheer. The only way really to know what you have is to test the product on the area where it's intended to be used.

■ A great many of the products on the market today are geared to skin type and say so plainly on the label. It makes picking the right one almost foolproof. If you have oily skin and pick a group of products formulated for oily skin you can be reasonably sure that the texture is compatible with your skin type. It takes a lot of the guesswork out of choosing. It can take some of the options away, too, since you may not find as much color choice in one line of special products as you might if you chose from various lines. That's why it's wise to know which formulations are best for your skin in addition to using those labeled "dry," "oily," or normal.

## Makeup Dos and Don'ts

DO avoid extremes—the bright sea-blue eye shadow, the bright red blush or lipstick. Aim for a subtle, natural look. DO take advantage of the "free" makeup sessions in stores, offered by most cosmetic companies from time to time. A trained makeup person will apply makeup and make suggestions for your skin and coloring. Although the consultation is free, you usually end up buying something.

DON'T forget that blending is probably the most important makeup step, no matter what kind of product you're using. It can keep you looking natural rather than artificial.

DON'T be fooled into thinking that makeup can cover up a poorly cared for skin. Makeup is great, but if it doesn't go on healthy skin, you're defeating its purpose.

DON'T give up if you're unhappy with the way your skin looks. Experiment with various cleansers, toners, etc. until you find a combination that agrees with your skin. If you have severe problems with breakouts, blackheads, excessively dry or oily skin, don't expect makeup to be the answer. A visit to a good dermatologist can help pinpoint the specific problem.

DO keep a makeup kit in your desk if you work outside your home. Refreshing your makeup during the day not only makes you look better, it gives you an emotional lift, too.

## BODY POLISH

It's perfectly possible to have the right clothes, makeup, and hair to make a positive impression, then blow it all anyway. Why? Because your body gives you away. Your body makes memorable statements about your insecurity, hostility, or whatever emotion you feel. Mannerisms, body language, or whatever you want to call the cluster

147

of gestures and body movements we all make are as important as what you say or how you look, yet you are probably least aware of them. Although you can look at yourself in the mirror, how often do you stand there and talk to yourself at length? You probably have very little idea of the kind of gestures you use in everyday circumstances and how they can give you away or help reinforce positively the image you want to project. To help you understand how important they are and how much they can convey, try this little experiment. Turn on your television and tune it to a drama or situation comedy. Now turn the sound down so you can't hear it. Watch the program for a few minutes and see how much you gather about what's happening just by watching the gestures and facial expressions. Turn the sound up every few minutes to check how accurate you've been. You'll find that the body language of the actors gave you a pretty good idea of what was going on. You could certainly tell whether the actors were angry, happy, frustrated, scheming, whatever, just by watching the expressions on their faces and how they moved their hands and bodies.

You reveal just as much about yourself with your gestures as these actors did. You will find that learning to read other people's body language and learning to control your own can make you a much more effective person.

## Interpreting the Signs

Most psychologists have observed similar gestures and bodily attitudes in similar circumstances. Body language seems to be so universal that Italians, French, Americans, and even Chinese and Japanese, who have very different cultural histories, seem to express themselves in surprisingly similar ways, though many nationalities do have a few typical gestures. Albert Mehrabian, an environmental psychologist whose color theories we talked about in a previous chapter, has done research in body language, too. He found that people show dominance, arousal, and pleasure by their body language. A relaxed stance or sitting position, he says, shows dominance and gives onlookers the message that you feel in control of the situation. A submissive attitude would be registered with a tense position, either sitting or standing. Extreme submissiveness is indicated by rigid body symmetry—think of the new recruit standing in front of the army sergeant. A tense body can also convey arousal—either pleasant or unpleasant. Eye contact, leaning forward toward another person, a head cocked attentively, all show a positive attitude toward another person.

Other researchers in the field point out that clenched fists or arms crossed on your chest show hostility or anger. "Open" gestures, gesturing with an open hand or hands, palms facing away or upward, sitting or standing so that your body appears open or receptive, are considered positive and a sign of sincerity by most people. Fidgeting, toe tapping, finger tapping, hair twisting and the like are signs of nervousness, boredom, or inattention.

The concept of private or personal space is closely allied to body language. In any situation, even one as temporary and unimportant as an elevator ride, we all establish a "private" space which, for the moment, we consider ours. Anyone who invades this space affects us, generally in a negative way, but not always. Invading someone's private space can sometimes be an effective intimacy technique. If you want to see how important this concept is, try this experiment. The next time you're having lunch with someone with whom you're not "best friends" or related to, try invading their half of the table. You might play with your water or wine glass, slowly pushing it around on the table until you have it on the other person's half of the table. Continue to move the glass as you chat and watch the other person. You will find that the person's attention is probably transferred

149

from what you're saying to what you're doing. He or she may register surprise, anxiety, discomfort, perhaps amusement, and if you continue, you may even be asked just what you think you're doing. In situations like this, we usually divide the table in half emotionally, or if there are several people at the table, we portion off the space around each diner. Anyone who intrudes on another's space is setting up a kind of negative tension. Even in a crowded bus or subway, we take a portion of the available space as ours and we range from uncomfortable to downright angry if someone intrudes on our space or bumps us. Psychologists have likened this behavior in us to the "territorial" instinct in animals. Most animals establish their territory and fight to keep or protect it. Your pet dog considers your house his territory and he will not willingly let another dog make himself comfortable without some amount of commotion.

In situations where you want to increase the degree of intimacy between you and another person, it's highly effective first to acknowledge the other person's territory or space, then insert yourself into it gently. You might edge closer to the other person as you talk encouragingly, you might even pat the other person's shoulder or maintain a high degree of eye contact. Moving in too much or too fast will usually be interpreted as hostility or at least as behavior that makes the other person uncomfortable.

Body language can be misleading if you concentrate on individual gestures. A single tense action or one show of hostility may not be meaningful, but when the gestures "cluster," or appear in groups, you can be certain they are expressing the predominant mood of the person using them. If someone you meet for the first time won't look you in the eye and shows very few overt signs of either pleasure, anger, or interest in your conversation, you can be fairly certain you're dealing with a cold fish. If, on the other hand, the person looks at you directly, smiles warmly and seems interested, but you notice that she is fidgeting with her handkerchief, you must weigh *all* the gestures to get a true reading. This is probably a warm, interested person who is a little shy on first meeting. Interpreting body language is not too different in this respect from interpreting spoken language. You must consider everything that is said, not just one remark, in order really to get the right perspective.

Let's talk about some specific instances to make this clearer. Jane entered her boss's office to report on a project she was working on. She walked in briskly—her brisk walk indicating her confidence—and sat down in the chair opposite her boss. Because her entrance was so brisk, and because she didn't hesitate even momentarily to check what the boss was doing and how responsive she might be to Jane's visit at this moment, Jane was setting up what could be negative tension. A moment's hesitation that showed some deference and indicated that she knew the other woman was boss, and by virtue of her position did not have to hear Jane out at this moment, would have been in order. As Jane began to talk and give her report, the boss crossed her arms in front of her chest and continued to sit this way, tapping her toe under her desk. In a situation such as this, the boss may feel guilty about not wanting to talk to Jane and decide to listen out of a sense of duty. Whatever Jane may be saying, however, is registered in a negative atmosphere. If Jane is wise, she'll recognize that she's in trouble here and try to get things into a more harmonious perspective. She could make some deferential remark, perhaps, "I'm sorry I barged in, but I felt it was important," or, "If you're terribly busy, I can come back another time." Responding to the boss's nonverbal clues could help Jane save the situation for herself and change the boss's attitude about the exchange.

In another kind of situation, Sarah is meeting her new mother-in-law-to-be for the first time. In addition to taking the time to dress in the way she feels is most appropriate for their luncheon meeting, Sarah sets the scene with her body language. She is careful to respect her mother-in-law's private space at the table. She sits in a relaxed but attentive way, with her head and upper torso leaning forward to show interest. She gestures with her hands open, palms raised and pointing away from her to indicate that she is sincere. She avoids tense, nervous fidgeting such as playing with the tablewear or twisting her napkin. Although she wants to seem relaxed, she sits erect enough to show respect for the other woman. These are very subtle gestures that are not difficult to master and that can contribute enormously to the total impression you create.

Just as moods are thought to be contagious—one or two persons in a "down" mood at a gathering can communicate that mood to the rest of the people there—body language and the feelings it represents are also thought to be contagious. Take this example: You are attending a school board meeting at which a sensitive issue is to be discussed. You feel tense and nervous and wonder what the outcome will be for your child so you sit with your legs pressed tightly together, hands clenched in your lap. After a few minutes, you notice that the woman sitting next to you is assuming a tense position. Before an "epidemic" of anxiety erupts, try to relax and see if you can't spread the more relaxed mood rather than reinforcing a tense one.

Body language is not the whole story; no single aspect of your image is, but it is a subtle and very meaningful part of you that may be overlooked if you don't give it some thought. Spend a little time observing people and how they signal their moods and feelings with their bodies and you'll begin to understand an entirely new language that you can put to work for yourself.

# 8
# How to solve your problem fashion and beauty situations

At *Glamour* we get thousands of letters every month from readers asking for advice on all kinds of problems. We've picked a few of the most typical questions to answer here so that you can solve some of the more specific dressing problems in your life. You'll find solutions for on-the-job problems, theater and restaurant problems, "black tie" problems, traveling problems, young-mother problems, figure problems, beauty problems.

## JOB INTERVIEWING

Q. *I am going to do a lot of full-scale job interviewing and I want to look professional. I cannot afford to buy a lot of clothes so I need some looks with versatility. What do you suggest?*

A. Invest in a suit or separates that look like a suit. Studies of personnel and business executives prove that the suit is the most successful thing a woman can wear for most kinds of job interviews. Pick a simple style—blazer-type jacket and soft skirt, something that's neither too full nor too slim. Pick a color that goes with other things in your wardrobe and you will find that you can mix both the jacket and skirt with other articles to give you several looks that will certainly see you through a lot of interviews. If your budget won't stretch to include a good suit (and quality matters here), buy a jacket that

154

works with several skirts you already own. This way you can create your own suit look. Under your jacket, wear a soft shirt in silk or a silky fabric. A shirt looks professional, but not stiff or rigid. A turtleneck sweater is another good choice if you're job hunting in cold weather.

## NEW OFFICE JOB

*Q. I have been raising my family, but now I am starting a new office job. I don't have many clothes that I feel are appropriate. What should I buy?*

A. Buy a minimum until you've been on the job for several weeks. Take a good look at what's being worn by women doing similar jobs and pick additional things you're sure will fit in. To start you off, consider these possibilities: a shirtwaist dress, a wrap dress, a skirt/ silk shirt/ jacket combination. They are all good choices for most settings unless your job requires specialized clothes or some sort of uniform. One jacket, two skirts that work with it, and two dresses should give you a good basic working wardrobe.

   Later, as you decide what else to add, remember that it's always best to "dress up" the professional ladder. Take note of what other women who have authority are wearing and dress as they do. In other words, dress as though you already have the job you aspire to.

## A FASHION LOOK

*Q. I am a copy supervisor at an advertising agency. How can I "edit" what's in fashion so that I look contemporary, yet not preoccupied witn clothes?*

A. Depending on what's in fashion at the moment, this can be tricky or simple. If current fashion runs to sexy, body-conscious clothes with deep slits or revealing lines,

155

you must choose with care. Anything that draws more attention to your body than your talent is going to get you the kind of attention you don't want. Since you work for an advertising agency in a creative department, you have greater flexibility than someone who works in a more conservative field—say an insurance company or a bank. Still, if you attend a conference or client meeting with a skirt that's slit so high you need to keep fussing with it, you're in trouble. If clothes are frilly and romantic and you arrive at the office in voluminous skirts and ruffles, again, you're in trouble because it's your clothes that are getting the attention, not you. You want clothes you're comfortable in, clothes that say you have an awareness of fashion (especially important in your field), yet you don't want to be considered a fashion groupie. Find the happy medium by asking yourself whether it's you or what you're wearing that dominates any given situation. If you must truthfully answer that what you're wearing is making the major impression, you've gone too far.

To look at it another way, you're usually safe if you add *one* fashionable piece to a basically classic look. If slim skirts with deep side slits are in fashion, you might team one with a very classic blazer and a classic silk shirt. You will present a polished appearance that says you know what's going on in the fashion world, yet you don't look like a fashion groupie.

## PACKING FOR TRIPS

Q. *I am a working woman who travels a lot on the job. My usual stay is overnight or a few days at most. How can I make dressing and packing for these trips easier? They often span climates—that is, to Florida where it's warm in January and then to New York where it's cold.*

A. A season-spanning jacket of lightweight wool or a wool and silk or rayon blend worn over a shirt and skirt

156

or a knit dress always look professional, are comfortable in many climates, and pack easily. If you wear the jacket, you can take a couple of shirts (a turtleneck for cooler weather), a knit dress, and you're set for a short business trip. If you go out in the evening, include a dressy blouse of some sort or a jersey dress. A velvet blazer works nicely for day and looks elegant in the evening. You will also find that knits of almost any kind are excellent travelers. They pack without wrinkling and are seasonless.

One trick many traveling women have discovered is the convenience of a garment bag as opposed to a conventional suitcase. One woman we know even packs for a two-week trip with one garment bag plus a carry-on. A garment bag can easily hold several days worth of clothes, and because the garments are on hangers, they aren't crushed as in a suitcase. A little tissue paper stuffed in shirt sleeves will keep them from wrinkling. You can hang one shirt over another on the same hanger; just button the top button to keep them from slipping around. Pants or skirts can usually be folded over a hanger and shirts hung on top of them to conserve hangers. Shoes, toilet articles, and a few other necessities can be packed in the carry-on bag. If your bags aren't too heavy to tote through the airport, you can often avoid having to check anything, saving yourself time.

## BUSINESS DINNERS

Q. *I often have to entertain clients for dinner in the evening. Since we usually have dinner in a good restaurant, I feel I should look elegant, but I want my clients to know I mean business, and I don't want to encourage any male/female relationships. What is appropriate on such occasions?*

A. You should look very much the way you do during the business day. A suit and a silk shirt or a velvet blazer, silk

157

shirt and skirt, a silky shirtdress or a wrap dress would all be appropriate. If you're worried about encouraging unwanted advances, remember that your attitude and the way you guide the conversation will set the tone of the evening. If you keep your conversation focused on business, with room for a few pleasantries, your intentions will be clear.

## CHANGEABLE TRAVEL CLIMATES

Q. *I travel on my job, often to places that could be warm or cool at any given time—such as Los Angeles and San Francisco and New Orleans. Although I check the weather before I go, it's no guarantee that the temperature won't change dramatically before or while I'm there. How can I solve this without arriving with two suitcases?*

A. Women who travel a great deal solve this problem by packing—and wearing—layers. First, wear or carry a trenchcoat. It's your top layer. The next layer is a blazer, which you should wear. If you know it's going to be coolish, add a turtleneck or some sort of sweater over a shirt and skirt or pants. If it's warmer, wear the blazer over a shirt. When you arrive, you can add the raincoat as another layer or peel it off. You can also peel off the jacket and use the raincoat to cover another temperature range. When the problem is whether it will be sweltering or just cool enough for a jacket, pack seasonless fabrics like cotton or synthetic knits and silk or silklike fabrics. Even tissue-weight wool gabardine is seasonless and can be worn in all but the hottest and most humid weather. Remember that knit dresses look marvelous under blazers —and they pack well. Natural fibers such as cotton, silk, and wool will wrinkle more than those combined with some synthetic.

# OFFICE TO FIELD

Q. *I am an engineer. My responsibilities include work in an office as well as almost daily visits to field sites. Often I must spend the morning in the office and the afternoon at sites, so I need clothes that are appropriate for both places. Can you help?*

A. Pants would seem to be an absolute necessity for you. For office wear, tailored pants with shirts or sweaters plus a jacket would be ideal. When you visit field sites, you might consider covering your office clothes with a loose-fitting washable top or some kind of heavy-duty industrial smock such as car mechanics or lab technicians wear. You might also slip a pair of loose coveralls over your office clothes.

# DRESSING FOR THE PUBLIC

Q. *I am just starting a law career and I'm very nervous about what to wear on my first court cases. Can you help?*

A. What you wear to some extent depends on your temperament. A classic suit of a neutral color, such as beige or gray, will make you look authoritative and serious. A suit is also comfortable to move around in if you have to get up and down, walking between judge and jury. If you feel you can handle more drama, some women lawyers have found that it's often an advantage to be a woman and to use your clothes to that effect. One highly successful lawyer likes to wear bright colors to court because she feels it makes her memorable—and she hopes, what she *says* more memorable. Unless you have a great deal of confidence in yourself and feel truly comfortable in court situations, it's best to play it safe at first, then adjust your style as you feel more comfortable.

## DINNERS AT HOME

Q. *I like to look festive when I'm entertaining people for dinner at home, but I do have to cook and I need something comfortable* and *practical. What can I wear?*

A. The fabric is more important than the style. Something that washes, rather than dry cleans is best. Some of the new synthetic silks look fabulous and they wash beautifully. A synthetic blend is also good. Slim, tapered pants with a soft shirt belted over them is a good choice. A long skirt with a soft shirt would also work. A caftan of some sort is another choice. If it's a casual party, you might even wear dressy jeans and a pretty shirt. There's nothing wrong with wearing an apron in the kitchen. This can make you feel less uptight about spilling things on yourself. The one thing to avoid is any kind of loose sleeve that gets into things—particularly the burner on your stove.

## IN THE PARK

Q. *I take my children to the park most afternoons and end up pushing them on the swings or crawling on the grass with them. I don't want to look a mess, but I usually do. Any suggestions?*

A. Nothing beats jeans for this kind of workout. A good-looking turtleneck sweater with a sweater jacket is ideal in cool weather; a T-shirt will be fine in warm.

## DINNER WITH HUSBAND

Q. *In addition to looking better, I know I feel a lot better if I can change into something more sophisticated when my husband comes home for dinner. I don't want to spend a lot for this part of my wardrobe since my major needs are durable, childproof daytime clothes. What can I buy?*

A. Rethink and rearrange your closet. Anything that you've worn all day or that you usually associate with the daily ritual of spills and tugs makes you feel less special. Sort your clothes into two groups: those that you wear during the day and those that you change into for "grown-up" evenings. Buy a pair of spiffy new jeans or casual pants, a jean or similar skirt, a couple of turtleneck sweaters and T-shirts and save them for "after-children" wear. Later, you can recycle them to daytime wear and since they are still casual and durable, they'll work. Washable, silklike shirts worn with casual pants or a skirt are a good choice for evening with your husband, and once in a while you might wear a caftan or skinny pants and a sexy top.

## PART-TIME JOB

Q. *I work part-time and I can't afford two wardrobes. I need something that's suitable for three days a week in an office and the rest at home, keeping my two-child household going. What will work for both?*

A. If you're really doing household chores at home, there's nothing that will work for this *and* the average office. You can, however, simplify your clothes life and keep your budget intact if you select your office clothes carefully. Make sure that *all* your office clothes work together in mood and color. Stick to a couple of basic colors and work around them. Start with a classic blazer and skirt and add shirts, sweaters, tailored pants, and a classic dress that can *all* be worn with your blazer. This way, every new addition will truly expand your wardrobe and what you have will be extremely versatile. As for what you wear at home, neat jeans and sweaters and T-shirts are unbeatable and represent no great expense.

## COMMUNITY ACTIVITIES

Q. *Now that my children aren't quite so dependent on me, I'm becoming more active in the community—going to political lunches, becoming active in groups supporting the women's movement. My present wardrobe of "house-bound" clothes needs expanding, but I'm on a budget. What will give me the most mileage for my money?*

A. Don't buy anything too trendy or geared to a particular occasion. Good classic clothes are timeless and go almost anywhere. A suit would be a great investment. Pick one in a neutral color that you can liven up with bright sweaters and blouses. Stick to a fairly classic style, perhaps a blazer-type jacket. An A-line skirt or a slim skirt with a kick pleat or a slit will endure for many seasons. Wear the suit alone in warm weather and under a coat in cold. Pick a color that works with other separates in your wardrobe; you will be able to mix the pieces of your suit with other things for several looks.

## COOL EVENING COVER-UPS

Q. *I have clothes to take me to the theater or restaurant with ease, it's what to wear over them that confuses me, especially when it's too warm for a coat but too cool to go out without one. Any ideas?*

A. A dressy jacket of some sort is ideal. There are some chenille blazers around now that make wonderful evening jackets. A velvet blazer is a classic that will also work. A sweater coat would be another sound choice. Pick a nubby or lacy texture in a good basic color such as beige, gray, or navy. This kind of cover-up is useful in both fall and spring and is always in style. A silk blazer is a nice luxury for over the shoulders in air-conditioned restaurants—if you can afford the luxury.

## "BLACK TIE" CHOICES

Q. *I am always at sea about what to wear when the invitation reads "black tie optional." Do I have to wear something long or can I wear a short dress?*

A. "Black tie optional" gives the men an out—they do not have to wear the formal black tie look, and you therefore don't have to wear a formal long dress. You can choose either a long or short one. If you feel too dressed up in something long, or if you don't have an appropriate long dress, by all means wear a short one. As a rule, short dresses far outnumber the long ones in such situations.

## SALES MEETINGS

Q. *My husband goes to sales meetings several times a year and wives are usually invited. There are usually days of sightseeing, big dinners, and a gala dance at the end of the trip. What would be appropriate to wear to these events?*

A. Let's take the activities one at a time. For daytime sightseeing, when you're apt to be in and out of tour buses and walking a lot, comfort is the key. A handsome pair of tailored pants with a sweater or a shirt, depending on the temperature, would be ideal. A casual skirt with the same tops would also work. Wear comfortable low to medium-heeled walking shoes. If you ruin your feet during the day, you won't enjoy the evening. A good silk shirt and a skirt with high-heeled strappy sandals and some pretty jewelry will work beautifully for most of the evening dinners. A crepe or silky dress will also work, but don't overdo the dressing up, you're likely to feel out of place. The wives of the executives usually set the dress tone for such occasions and you'll discover most won't overdo it. For the gala, do wear something long if you have it. You'll find that most women tend to opt for long dresses at this kind of party. The safest choice is a long slip dress—one with a camisole top and shoestring straps is always appropriate. You could also wear a camisole top and long skirt of some kind, maybe a slim one with a deep slit at the side or in front. Stay away from the "prom dress" look or anything too fussy. A simple, elegant look is what you're after.

## DINNERS WITH CLIENTS

Q. *My husband must entertain clients for dinner in the evening. The clients' wives are usually invited, too. I never know what to wear. I don't want to be too dressed up and intimidate the other women and I don't want to look too casual and have it appear that I don't care about the evening. What's appropriate?*

A. Since the people you are entertaining are clients of your husband, your main goal should be to put them at ease. If you overdress, you will obviously make the other women feel uncomfortable. A suit with a dressy blouse or a camisole in a silky fabric would be especially pretty, would look pulled-together yet not be off-putting. An elegant silk dress in a simple style such as a shirtwaist, would also be appropriate. Don't wear a long skirt or dress. It looks inappropriate in a restaurant setting.

## A LARGE BOSOM

Q. *I am a very large-bosomed woman. Can I wear the new wide-shouldered look?*

A. Yes, within reason. Extremes in padded shoulders will make you look top-heavy, but gentle padding through the shoulders will help balance the size of your bosom and actually be quite flattering. It's the small-bosomed woman who really has trouble with padded shoulders. Their width makes her bosom look even smaller. If you find something you like very much but feel there's too much shoulder padding, don't be afraid to remove the pads and replace them with smaller ones. Any dime store or notions department carries a selection of shoulder pads you can pick from, so it's an easy task. Most pads can actually be pinned into the shoulder seam of your garment, so you don't even have to do any sewing!

# A SHORT WAIST

Q. *Wide wrapping belts seems to be part of the look of many new clothes. I am short waisted. Can I wear these belts?*

A. If you wear one, pick the narrowest. A really wide one will make you look as though you have almost no upper torso. The best choice for you is a very soft wrap belt not more than two inches wide. You'll have the look of a wrap, but since the belt is soft, it will crush down a bit and you won't look as though you have no waist.

# FULL HIPS

Q. *Skirts have slimmed down and my hips haven't. I would really like to try the narrower look, but I'm afraid I'll pick the wrong thing. What would be best for me?*

A. Don't pick the slimmest of slim skirts. Try on those that have some softening through the waist and hip— tucks, gathering, or side-slash pockets for ease. After trying on several, you should be able to find at least one that looks well on you. You can also try slim dresses with the same detailing. They should work nicely, too.

## TOO THIN

Q. *I am very slender and have always been glad a layered look was in. Now that clothes are narrowing down a bit, I'm dismayed. I don't want to look pathetic, but I don't want to look out of style, either.*

A. Layered dressing is still in and always will be, because it functions so well in many situations and climates. Still, you don't have to count yourself out on narrow clothes. If you'd like to try a slim skirt, look for one with shirring or a few darts at the waist or hip and look for some kind of slit that will show the curve of your calf. This softens the angular look of a perfectly straight skirt. You can also wear a slim skirt with a large, soft sweater or shirt on top. If you pick a top that's worn on the outside and that hits you at hip level, it will soften the look of your thinness considerably. Stay away from slim, clingy dresses. There's no way you're not going to look like a beanpole in them.

## SMALL FRAME

Q. *I am short, five feet, and slender, ninety-eight pounds. I look fragile and also young for my age, but I have a responsible job and find it difficult to get people to take me seriously. I want them to know I'm the boss, not the secretary. How can I dress my small frame with more authority?*

A. You need to dress with an eye to adding more stature in addition to picking polished, pulled-together clothes. First of all, a monotone looks well, gives a longer line. If you wear separates, keep top and bottom in the same color family. Don't wear wide or contrasting belts, they will break the line and make you appear even shorter. If you wear a belt, make it a very narrow one. You will find that hard-edged fabrics such as gabardine, poplin, broadcloth, certain types of corduroy, and twills have the au-

166

thority and polish that softer fabrics such as crepe, satin, silk, and velour don't. Neutral colors such as beige, gray, navy, maroon, and deep bottle green also help add authority.

When picking styles, lean to the more severe rather than fussy or little-girl looking clothes. Avoid ruffles, lace, too many gathers and pastel colors. One good look for you would be a beige sweater jacket over a deeper beige silk shirt and slim beige skirt with a kick pleat. Keep your shoes and stockings in the same tone as your skirt.

## PROBLEMS WE OFTEN HEAR ABOUT

### Oily Hair

Q. *I have a husband, two small children, a very busy job, and extremely oily hair. I simply don't have time to fuss much with my hair, yet if I don't wash it almost daily, it looks terrible. What do you suggest?*

A. Cut your hair as short as is flattering to you. If your hair is curly, have it cut in a soft, curly cap style. If it's straight, have it cut so that it curves close to your head, perhaps with some kind of bangs to soften the shortness. Bangs and brushed-back sides are becoming and look contemporary. Either of these ideas allows you to wash your hair daily and blow it dry quickly. It should take no more than twenty minutes from start to finish for either look, and that's about as little time as you can expect to spend on a hair routine. If your hair is blond or no darker than medium brown, buy a dry shampoo and use it on those days when you just can't wash your hair.

### Baby-Fine Hair

Q. *My hair is fine and I had a permanent to give it body, but this only made things worse. My hair looks frizzy and*

167

*I can't do much with it. Help!*

A. Fine hair is the most difficult to permanent successfully. Unless it's done with great care, you end up with frizz. For now, condition your hair with a deep-conditioning treatment product every two weeks and begin having the permanent trimmed off. The more you can trim off, the more control you'll have over your hair and the more manageable it will become. Once you're rid of the permanent, don't have another. Try to have your hair cut in a simple style not more than chin length. If you don't know how to blow it dry successfully, ask your hairdresser to show you. A good cut and good blow-dry technique should make you master of your hair.

## Pale Skin, Lashes, Everything

Q. *I have exceedingly fair skin, pale lashes and brows, and without makeup, I look like a ghost. I'm afraid to use too much makeup for fear of overdoing it. What would be a good makeup routine for me?*

A. Mascara, blush, and lipcolor are the essentials. Spend most of your makeup time on your eyes, applying several coats of dark brown mascara to both your top and bottom lashes. This will look natural if you let the mascara dry between coats and run a clean lash brush through your lashes after every coat. You might also try a light coat of mascara on your brows to provide some emphasis. If you have time, a soft brown or gray shadow applied to lids would also add some drama. Use a coral or tawny blush on cheeks. Powder blush is probably easiest to control because you can easily brush off any excess. Keep your lip color in the same color family as your blush. Pick a lipstick with a sheer, shiny texture for the most natural look.

168

## Dramatic Looks

Q. *I am a brunette with dramatic coloring. I don't want to avoid makeup completely, but I always feel I look overdone. What can I do?*

A. Pick the softest colors in the tones you feel flatter you most—pink, peach, or tawny. Use this tone on your cheeks and lips. A color with a bit of frosting—not the heavy sparkly stuff—but something with just a bit of shimmer in it, will give you the most natural look. Instead of mascara on brows and lashes, try brushing them with a little petroleum jelly to add shine but not a heavy, unnatural look. If you want to use eyeshadow, pick something with a bit of life—a russet, a soft mauve, or smoky gray—and apply the color with the lightest strokes. Either powder or cream will work.

## Bushy Hair

Q. *My hair is so coarse and bushy I can't do a thing with it. What will help control it?*

A. A good cut is a must. A short cut works for some face shapes. Chin to shoulder length uses the weight of your hair to help pull it down and control it. You will also find that a cream rinse used after every shampoo will make your hair behave better. Deep-condition it every three or four weeks to keep the ends in shape.

## Skin Breakouts

Q. *I have recently taken a new job that puts considerable pressure on me. Ever since I've started, I've had trouble with my skin. It breaks out and it's never done this before. What is causing this problem? What can I do about it?*

A. You are probably suffering from what some dermatologists are beginning to call "working women's acne."

169

More and more women are turning up in dermatologists' offices complaining of breakouts when they have no history of them during their adolescence. Most dermatologists feel the condition is due to stress. Stress affects basic hormone balance and eventually can cause skin to erupt and break out. If the condition is severe and persists, see a dermatologist. If you feel it's not necessary to see a doctor, ask your pharmacist to recommend a good drying lotion to use on the breakouts. Avoid using any oily makeup products on your skin while the condition exists. Eat a well-balanced diet and get adequate sleep. Above all, try to relax a bit more and take your job in stride. Think carefully about the real priorities in your life and give up those that take up your time but aren't high on your priority list.

Although you are probably suffering from acne, no one but your doctor can rule out the possibility of an allergy. If acne medications don't help or if your breakouts look more like a rash or hives than pimples, check with a dermatologist. It's usually not possible to treat allergic skin conditions successfully with over-the-counter medications.

## CHANGING NEIGHBORHOODS

Q. *I am moving from a very "collegiate" sort of neighborhood to a more sedate and proper one. I know I can't go out in my grubby jeans all the time, but I don't want to get dressed up to go to the supermarket. What's appropriate for running errands and being out and about?*

A. Don't assume you can't wear jeans anymore. If you wear freshly pressed jeans with a good-looking shirt or sweater and a jacket or coat of some sort, you will look perfectly fine. It's the rumpled, unpressed look you want to avoid.

## IMAGE CHANGE

Q. *I have recently gotten a job promotion and am now in charge of several women who used to be—and still are—close friends. I need help establishing my new "boss image." What will do it?*

A. It's important for you to remember that you will probably have to put some emotional distance between you and your friends in order to make a boss–employee situation work. Clothes will help. Try to wear the most polished looks you have—dress-and-jacket combinations, suits or suit looks. Add as much polish as you can in the way of accessories—a scarf at your neck, a bit of gold jewelry. If your job necessitates handling a lot of papers, carry a briefcase—even though it's empty most days. No one will know what's inside but you.

## TRAVEL CLOTHES

Q. *I am taking my first trip to Europe, where I will be visiting mostly large cities such as Paris and Rome. I plan to attend as many evening cultural events such as opera, concerts and the theater (I understand French) as I can. I know what I'm going to wear during the day, but what is appropriate for evening?*

A. You'll find that most Europeans tend to dress a little more in the evening than Americans. You'll see more "dressy" clothes in both restaurants and theaters. Since you'll be on the move and aren't likely to see the same people twice, you don't need variety, so clothes should not be a problem. A dark-colored slip dress or a camisole and skirt worn under a dressy jacket—perhaps a velvet blazer—would be a perfect look. Another choice would be a silk shirtdress of some sort. Strap sandals will dress up your look perfectly.

171

## HAIR PROBLEM

Q. *I feel my clothes work well for my lifestyle and I also feel confident that they look "quality." Still I often feel unhappy with my appearance. I think it's because I have very fine hair, which is oily. It seems to be lank and unattractive most of the time. What can I do to perk it up a bit?*

A. This is difficult—but not impossible—hair. You must resign yourself to washing it at least every other day to keep it shiny and bouncy looking. Since this is time-consuming, you should have a short, simple cut. Look back to pages 140 and 141 (where hairstyles are sketched) and consider something close to the short cuts there. Bangs usually swept to one side, add softness to short styles. A curling iron would be a good investment for you. One of the new ones with steam or even little teeth to hold the hair will give you extra body and control. Stay away from shampoos with thickening additives. They will make your hair appear greasy faster.

## MATERNITY CLOTHES FOR A SHORT WOMAN

Q. *I am pregnant and short—just five feet. I know I am going to have a problem as I grow. I look so overwhelmed by the full maternity clothes. What can I wear that will be flattering to me?*

A. Go back to Chapter 1 and review the advice for short women. Much of it will still work for you now. Stay away from two-piece maternity clothes as much as possible and if you do wear them, pick only those that are the same color top and bottom so you don't cut your height in half by wearing two different colors. Stick to the slimmest styles; those with fullness starting close to the waist, rather than from a yoke at the bosom, will be best. Deep colors will help elongate your body. It's very important to keep your stockings in the same color family as your clothes now. This, too, will help elongate your body. For the same reason, pants would be good for you now. They give a nice long line. If you're usually slim and not over-weight, you'll probably find you can get by with regular clothes for quite a while. Some women manage it for six months. You might try drawstring pants and dresses with drawstring waists. These can often be worn by pregnant women during the first five or six months of pregnancy. Most of all, don't focus too much on your height. Enjoy the pleasure of being pregnant and of planning for your new baby. You'll forget all about how out of proportion you felt once the baby arrives.

# 9
# Conclusion: Putting it all together

To put together all the information in this book so that it works for you, you have to become aware of where you are at this point in your life and what's appropriate for you. You must know enough about what kind of clothes you feel comfortable in and what effect they will have on others—and on you. Once you have mastered this, you will be able to take your good basic knowledge and move it from one area of your life to another and to make it grow and change with you.

As a final thought in this book, here are the stories of two women who didn't do it right at first, but finally learned, as you can too, to make your fashion identity a lifetime asset.

Karen was bright and pretty and had been working in an advertising agency for three years. When she first started working, she was one of a dozen young women with similar jobs. Each wanted to be noticed so that she could be singled out to be moved up. Each had her own way of trying to make herself stand out. For Karen, it was dressing with a great deal of creativity, sometimes so much so that her look was a little outrageous, but because she was in a creative department it worked—other creative people noticed her. She was recognized for her flair and her ideas and she was promoted. But soon she began accompanying account executives on client visits. Karen's job changed, but her look didn't. She began to get negative feedback about her clothes from superiors until finally her immediate superior, a sympathetic woman only a few years older than Karen, pulled her aside and told her that she had to stop dressing so conspicuously if she were going to advance and have contact with the agency's clients.

What Karen had been doing was to continue to define her needs by goals that were no longer appropriate. Her old image had worked, it had got her noticed and promoted, but now her needs were different. She had to change, to shift her thinking into a more conservative look that wouldn't be off-putting to many kinds of clients, from bankers to car dealers. If Karen has a good sense of herself and of what she likes and what works in various circumstances, she will be able to change her thinking and pull together a slightly different kind of look. She did, and she did it in a way that was virtually foolproof. She looked around her and noticed what her boss wore, what other women on the way up were wearing, and she started dressing the way they did. She still likes to have a sense of adventure in her clothes and she always manages to wear something that makes her feel true to her own identity—an art deco print scarf, a piece of beautifully designed but off-beat jewelry—yet she looks perfectly appropriate for the job she is doing.

Mary had a different kind of problem, but the source of it is similar to Karen's and perhaps to some problems you may be having, too. Mary had married just out of college and had a child a year or so later. Most of her wardrobe consisted of things she had owned in college and for the most part were suitable during the day when her needs were for casual clothes that could take a beating. When Mary went out on an occasional evening with her husband and friends, she pulled out a dress or skirt and shirt she'd worn in college for dates. She didn't feel particularly spiffy, but she felt her look would "do." It did—for a while. Mary's first clue that something was wrong with her image came in an experience with a baby sitter. She hired a sixteen-year-old girl to sit with her son several times. "Usually it was just for a couple of hours in the afternoon while I shopped," said Mary. But one day, Mary needed a sitter for an entire Saturday, while she and her husband visited friends in another town. Mary told the sitter that she could have her date over to watch television in the evening if she wanted, and left a number where she could be reached. When she and her husband arrived home about 10:00 P.M., a little earlier than they'd planned, they were greeted by a living room full of sixteen-year-olds dancing and eating *their* refrigerator bare. Mary was furious. "I thought I told you to have your boyfriend over to watch TV," she said, "not to treat the neighborhood to a disco party." The sitter responded that she didn't think Mary would care about the party because Mary probably did a lot of discoing herself. It was a weak excuse and didn't make Mary feel any better about the sitter's lack of consideration. But this, combined with several other experiences she had with other sitters who didn't take her requests very seriously, made Mary begin to realize that she commanded no authority with the sitters. She was regarded as almost a teenager herself.

Everything came to a head when Mary wanted to be elected to a local school board office. She would be good at the job, she knew, but people just didn't seem to take her seriously when she said she could do it. She made a few speeches, talked to other people in the community, but she lost the election by a landslide to another woman only a couple of years her senior.

Mary was terribly disappointed and she tried to figure it all out over lunch in the city with an old friend. Her friend told Mary to look at what she was wearing to their lunch —which was in a good restaurant in a very large city. Mary was wearing a plain crew-neck sweater, a pleated skirt, low-heeled walking shoes, and patterned knee socks. She looked sixteen, more like a student than a young mother lunching with a friend in the city. Then Mary noticed what her friend, who was the same age and also a full-time mother was wearing. She had on a silk shirt, a softly gathered skirt, and a blazer. She was wearing stockings and suede pumps. "Who do you think the waiter will give the check to?" Mary's friend asked with a laugh. Mary got the point.

She began replacing her collegiate wardrobe with a more grown-up one. This didn't mean throwing out all her old clothes and spending a great deal of money on new ones. It did mean buying a few things—a dressy shirt, some shoes, and a couple of dresses to wear when she needed to present a more authoritative appearance.

Like Karen, Mary's life had changed, but her image remained the same. If you're really aware of the image you should create to achieve your present goals and how to project that image through your clothes, you're home free. You have an understanding of fashion and image that will stay with you a lifetime and will work for rather than against you as you grow and change.

Take a look at the ten questions here. How you answer them can reveal how much of a sense of self you have and how well you understand the function of clothes in your life.

1 Is what you wear in keeping with what's worn by other successful people around you—in the office, at school, in your community?

2 Do you usually feel comfortable and at ease with what you wear?

3 Do you give a reasonable amount of thought to organizing your looks rather than just letting them happen?

4 Do you occasionally offer some surprises and freshness in your looks rather than being the same old predictable you?

5 Do you usually know what you're going to wear for various occasions, and do you own appropriate things?

6 Are you able to get dressed and out or on with your day most of the time instead of standing in front of your closet feeling insecure?

7 Do you feel people take you seriously when you want them to?

8 Does your appearance make you feel good about yourself most of the time?

9 When you look great, do you feel you planned it that way rather than that you "got lucky"?

10 Do you feel emotionally able to change your look when your life changes?

If you can answer yes to most of these questions, you're well on your way to developing a good fashion identity that will be flexible enough to stay with you indefinitely, no matter what the situation. If you had to answer no to more than three of them, you could do with another reading of this book. The answers are all here, you just have to learn to put them together in a way that makes sense for .

you

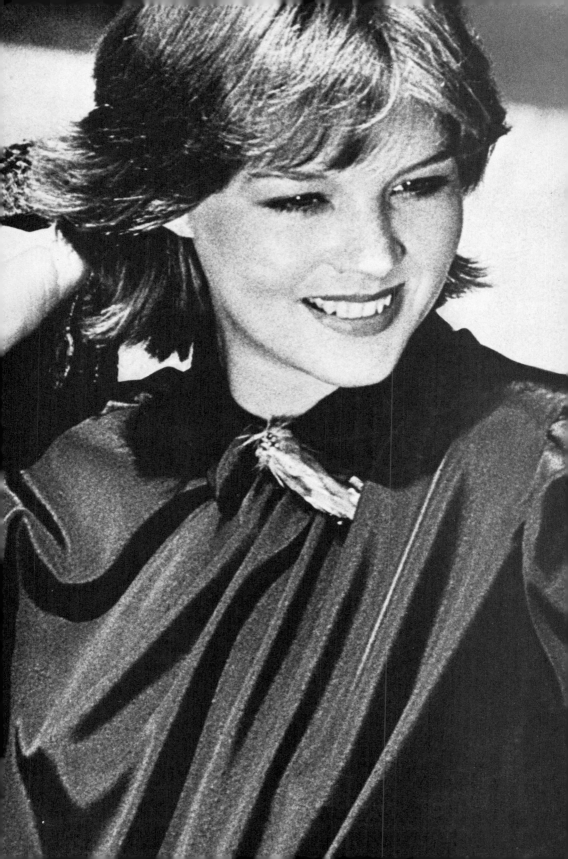

# INDEX

185

# Index